CHAKRA MEDITATION

Layne Redmond

CHAKRA MEDITATION

Transformation
through the
Seven Energy Centers
of the Body

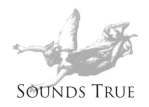

SOUNDS TRUE

Sounds True, Inc., Boulder CO 80306

Published 2004
Printed in Korea

ISBN 1-59179-178-2

Other Sounds True Titles By Layne Redmond
Chakra Breathing Meditations
Invoking the Muse
Chanting the Chakras: The Roots of Awakening

TABLE OF CONTENTS

Color plates follow page 42

Introduction

IN 1969, when I was sixteen years old, my best friend's aunt gave me *Yoga, Youth and Reincarnation* by Jess Stearn. Having been trained as a dancer, I could easily fit my body into the *yoga* postures illustrated in the book, and I enjoyed the exhilarated state generated by the breathing exercises. Within a year, I found the first of my many yoga teachers and soon read *Be Here Now* by Ram Dass, working my way through the list of transformational books he recommended. As a teenager I was struggling with the perennial questions of "Why are we who we are?" and "If we are not satisfied with who we are and how our lives are unfolding, what can we do about it?" The path of yoga and meditation led me to look for the answers to these questions within myself. Yoga teaches us that our minds are aspects of the infinite, eternal, creative consciousness of the universe, and gives us the tools to remove the illusions and confused ideas that prevent us from realizing this sacred truth. There is no greater treasure than knowing ourselves, and no greater gift than to learn the techniques that will enable us to do this. It is very exciting to have the opportunity to pass on some of the incredible practices I have learned over the past 35 years from my teachers.

The wisdom developed through thousands of years of yoga practice and contained within this book and guided CD will give you powerful tools to understand how your mind functions, and how and why you create the relationships and situations that exist in your life. You will begin to understand what is stopping you from reaching your fullest potential, and how to prevent the loss of your mental, emotional, and intellectual energy to negative situations and unhealthy interactions with others. You will learn how to develop your own inner sources of creativity and personal power, enabling you to transcend patterns of behavior that hold you back. Yoga helps to clear away your misconceptions about who you are, and helps you understand how social, cultural, and familial bonds keep you from seeing the true depths of your spiritual being.

This integrated book and CD learning program focuses on the electromagnetic infrastructure of the mind and body known in yoga as the *chakras*. For centuries the mystics, scholars, and yogis of India have explored, mapped out, and created techniques for working with the dimensions of consciousness contained within the chakras. These time-tested and proven methods provide effective ways to open, balance, and awaken the chakras, enhancing the evolution of human awareness. This process is equivalent to rewiring the nervous system to handle higher voltages and more powerful currents of awareness. The practices included in this program are easy to learn, invigorating, and extremely powerful, producing peace of mind, improved physical health, and spiritual growth.

The first two chapters of the book provide an overview of the seven chakras and how they function. The following seven chapters explore in depth the realms of information embodied in each chakra. Each chapter includes instruction on the use of the geometric image of the chakra, the *yantra*. This is a power diagram of wholeness and integration that tunes you into the deepest spiritual dimensions of the chakra.

Chapter Ten details the specific instructions for the breathing, visualization, and chanting practices on Tracks One through Seven on the enclosed CD. Please be sure to read the brief description of each practice before listening to the recording. The seventh practice on the CD is a traditional purification meditation that opens, clears, and balances the chakras, awakening the powerful life force residing at the base of the spine. This awakened energy further activates the chakras, sweeping you into new dimensions of experience and awareness. Your state of consciousness determines what your life experiences will be, and as consciousness expands, your understanding of every aspect of life will also. The final chapter is a short overview of the lineage of yoga teachers that have passed this information down to us over the last 5,000 years. I have also included a list of resource books for those who wish to learn more.

This program offers the energy practices that underlie my work as a creative artist. They are the source of my inspiration and creativity, and have brought me success as a performer, recording artist, and author. Commitment and consistency in pursuing these techniques will give you the means for connecting to the ultimate and highest source of your own being. You will have more clarity about the purpose of your life, and the necessary tools to help you pursue the path you choose. May this be the beginning of a spiritual transformation that will sustain you for the rest of your life. ☀

CHAPTER
ONE

The Seven Dimensions of Reality

SINCE THE BEGINNING of time, wisdom traditions have told us there are seven heavens, seven planes of experience, or seven dimensions of consciousness that we must journey through to enter into the totality of our luminous awakened Self. This sacred, realized, essential, eternal, or higher Self is the deepest core of our consciousness that is in touch with the creative source of all life. The total or true Self directly experiences its primal connection with everything, and is conscious of the unity and structure of creation. The renowned psychotherapist, Carl G. Jung, spoke of the archetype of the higher Self as the blueprint for all of humanity as well as for each individual human being. This blueprint of the mind's infinite potential is waiting in the depths of our unconscious to be brought forth into the world. As the blueprint unfolds, the force of the awakening Self inspires, motivates and guides our evolution into higher dimensions of awareness.

This archetypal journey is an internal, spiritual passage through the dimensions of our own consciousness that shifts our sense of identity away from the social or personal self (focused on the physical body and our individual mind) to this sacred Self. The yogic tradition details this journey through seven spheres of energy and information known as the *chakras*. The word *chakra* comes from Sanskrit, the ancient language of India, and translates as "circle," "wheel," or "vortex of energy." The chakra system is the electromagnetic structure of our consciousness, created by the flow of our life force through the mind and body. The chakras are the intersections of energy and consciousness located along the main energy channel flowing from the upper brain to the base of the spine, and regulating our physical, mental, and emotional states.

Each chakra represents a realm of thoughts, emotions, desires, goals, and ideals. The first chakra at the base of the spine is concerned with physical survival. Moving up the spine, the second chakra in the lower abdomen is concerned with relationships, the third chakra at the navel with our place in the world, the fourth chakra at the heart center with the power of compassion and love, the fifth chakra at the throat with the power of communication of ideas of truth and beauty, the sixth chakra in the center of the brain with the power of meditative and cognitive awareness, and the seventh chakra at the crown of the head with the realization of our spiritual Self. The process of awakening the chakras and moving our awareness up from the first chakra to the seventh chakra is our journey back to the infinite potential of the highest Self.

If the flow of our life energy and consciousness is blocked at any point within the chakras or the channels through which the energy flows to the chakras, this will have a profound effect on our physical and mental health, how we see ourselves and others, how we operate in the world, and our ability to manifest our highest potential. In this program you will learn what causes blockages in the chakras and how to open, balance, and activate them, bringing the energetic system of the mind and body to an optimal state of functioning.

We perceive reality through the chakra in which our awareness is most habitually concentrated. In most cases, our awareness is usually fixated in the first, second, or third chakras, or dispersed among those three. Located at the base of the spine, the first chakra, *Muladhara*, is where all the vast potential of our life force lies coiled and waiting to be awakened. The activation of this energy through yoga practices is the beginning of the evolutionary journey through the chakras.

Muladhara is the root center of physical experience and the instinctive issues and fears of this chakra revolve around security, food, and shelter—the fundamental concerns of biological survival. Psychologically, the first chakra is a self-centered place.

Here we are concerned with our own thoughts and feelings, sometimes to the point of neglecting those around us. The world appears as a reality to be conquered, controlled, acquired, and hoarded. Our survival and possessions come first, and we identify with the money and material things we accumulate. Unbalanced first chakra issues arising from insecurities about our basic needs are often the driving forces behind jealous and violent behavior.

Anxieties and fears surrounding the ability to provide for life's necessities can easily take over the mind. Fear of the future, low self-esteem, diminished vitality, and depression characterize an unenergized or unbalanced first chakra. Deep-seated insecurities about the future and the present lead us to feel that the world is not safe and that we must protect ourselves and what we have from outside enemies. First chakra fears are frequently used to keep us within accepted norms. If we announce that we are going to pursue our dreams rather than maintain the status quo, family and friends often quickly warn, "You will end up alone and broke." More dreams are abandoned due to first chakra fears than anything else.

Protecting family, home, and food supply from outsiders has always been a central issue that societies have to address. History is often the story of one group taking exactly those things away from another group, so the concerns are extremely valid. Yet leaders on every level, from the family to the government, often seize on less-than-conscious first chakra issues to frighten, polarize, and gain control of others.

An activated and well-functioning first chakra enables us to detach from identifying the self with material reality. We can make sure that we have what we need, but we no longer define ourselves by what we have. As the Muladhara chakra is energized and balanced, we gain a security that is not related to the material world. We become much less susceptible to control by others through first chakra fears. Security is a state of consciousness. If we feel secure within ourselves, we are able to meet whatever life brings us with serenity, knowing that we can take care of ourselves or seek appropriate help to survive.

Sexual energy, fantasy, pleasures, and desires for relationships dominate our awareness at the second chakra, *Svadisthana*, located in the pelvic region. The main motivation of the second chakra is to make sure desires are satisfied. Seeking pleasure through food, drink, drugs, and sexual encounters can become a mesmerizing obsession.

Svadisthana's negative qualities—lust, anger, greed, delusion, pride, and envy—develop from a sense of possessiveness. These emotions arise as a result of trying to maintain control over people and things that are sources of pleasure. As the second chakra comes into balance, we can detach from these emotions, avoiding the disturbances they cause. Rather than concentrating on others as sources of fulfillment, we shift the focus to ourselves and our creativity, freeing up energy for intellectual and artistic pursuits. An illuminated second chakra often produces artists, poets, musicians, writers, dancers, or inventors.

Svadisthana chakra, the seat of the collective and individual unconscious, acts as a storehouse of karma, past lives, and the effects of our experiences in this life. It is the primary repository of the *samskaras*, the conditioned patterns of response that drive our behavior.

The samskaras can be understood as the personality patterns we inherit at birth along with the conditioning process that occurs as life unfolds. Each action, thought, emotion, and experience we have leaves a subtle impression that shapes our consciousness. Many of these impressions get pushed into forgetfulness by the continuing unfolding of our life, but they leave residues of their consequences in the mind. These subconscious imprints color all of our responses, states of mind, emotions, attitudes, and expressions of character, causing us to act and respond in certain set patterns of behavior. The samskaras are responsible for many of the blockages in our chakra energy system.

Yoga practices serve to remove this habitual world from the mind and the blockages in our consciousness by dissolving the samskaras. Practicing yoga, meditation, and *pranayama* (rhythmic breathing exercises) creates new, beneficial routines that clear the subconscious, promote clarity, and allow the free flow of energy through the chakras. It becomes easier to avoid old cycles of emotional turmoil, freeing energy to create new, positive patterns of behavior that bring contentment and peace.

Instinctive territorial and dominance drives come strongly into play at the *Manipura* chakra, found at the solar plexus. We see these innate behaviors in many species around us. In nature, territory must be defined and defended to ensure survival. Yet we can become conscious of these drives and harness them in a balanced way without becoming domineering or being dominated. Balancing the issues and energies of this chakra allows us to learn how to set and respect healthy boundaries.

Fire and intellect dominate the third chakra personality, who moves toward personal goals—without always considering the consequences—in an extremely competitive, assertive, and courageous manner. When the unbridled passions of this chakra dominate, family and friends can be sacrificed in the intense push to gain power, respect, and recognition. Out-of-balance Manipura energy can result in a person willing to wipe out the competition to achieve his or her ends. Control of others is maintained through the threat of anger, vengeance, and violence. Carl G. Jung noted, "We still have to be polite to people to avoid the explosions of Manipura."[1] There is never enough fame, fortune, power, and command over others and the physical environment to satisfy the out-of-control third chakra personality.

Most of us, including the world's political leaders, have been operating from the first three chakras' fears and concerns for thousands of years. To transcend these life-threatening—indeed planet-threatening—modes of behavior, we must become aware of how underlying fears rule our lives, keep us within safe and acceptable social norms, and prevent us from connecting to the sacred Self. It is essential to raise our conscious awareness up from the lower three chakras into the fourth chakra, the heart chakra.

When we reach the heart chakra, *Anahata*, the seat of the higher emotions of love, compassion, kindness, and empathy, we set foot on a powerful spiritual path. Consciously centering our energy, thoughts, and actions in the heart helps us transcend the lower chakra issues that could mesmerize us forever. Realized teachers have always taught that compassion and lovingkindness for all beings is the path to liberation. As we dissolve any blockages to unconditional love, the journey into the upper chakras begins.

The fifth chakra, *Vishuddha*, is situated in the region of the throat. This chakra's power is to verbalize and communicate information received from all of the other chakras. As the ruler of the organs of speech, a purified and activated throat chakra gives an inspiring authority and beauty to the voice. The power of communication in the fifth chakra also allows us to receive and understand information from our dream states. When awareness rises to this chakra, we experience simplicity of thought, detachment, and serenity. The motivating desire is for solitude in which to meditate.

The sixth chakra, *Ajna*, found at the top of the spine in the middle of the brain, represents the highest expansion of intellectual powers and meditative states of awareness. This seat of intuition and clairvoyance knows the past, present, and future. The only remaining desire is for complete union with the ultimate awareness of the seventh dimension of consciousness, the *Sahasrara*.

As the life force is awakened at the first chakra, the transformational fountain of energy rising up through each of the chakras culminates in the sparkling union of the individual self with the source of infinite consciousness at the seventh plane, the Sahasrara. Not actually a chakra, but often referred to as one, Sahasrara, experienced at the crown of the head, is the source of all reality. The chakras as energy matrixes belong to the realm of the mind and body. This center is the mediating point between the mind/body and higher realities. At the Sahasrara, the socially conditioned self-image of the ego dissolves completely into the primordial awareness of the eternal sacred Self.

A 1,000-petaled lotus symbolizes this transcendental union with the infinite intelligence of the universe. The Sahasrara is formless and with form, yet untouched by form, beyond form. It is everything, and it is nothing. At this level of consciousness, the illusion that one is an individual entity fades into the knowledge that all things are aspects of the One. As a result of the unification of the chakras with the source of creation, all desires dissolve into an extending, unbounded state of awareness. In the yogic tradition, this state is traditionally known as *nirvana* or the Realized Self.

To begin this journey, we will study the issues and energies of each chakra. We will learn traditional yoga practices to clear our minds, balance the energies in the chakras, and begin to raise our awareness to higher levels. These practices remove energetic obstacles and blockages, shifting our sense of identity from the personal self to the eternal Self. The resulting free flow of energy dissolves the troubling and repressed memories of the past, cleansing the mind of anxiety and tension. The tissues and cells of the body and brain are transformed and revitalized, creating a radiant mind and body. Intuition increases, along with a heightened understanding of the subtle forces that structure reality, enabling us to make better decisions. Feelings of satisfaction and serenity increase, and we develop a sense of quiet detachment from the whirl of everyday events. We move ever closer to union with the imperishable, innermost Self. ✿

CHAPTER
TWO

The Power Structure of the Chakra System

AT THE END of the 19th century, spiritual practices from India known as *yoga* were introduced to the West. Yoga, a practical science of self-development, has been evolving for at least 5,000 years. The word *yoga* comes from the root *yuj*, meaning to join, yoke, or unite the mind's attention to the supreme state of primordial awareness, the source of the innermost Self. The goal of yoga is to clear the mind so that we can actually understand who we are and what our purpose in life is.

While there are many different yoga traditions, Westerners are most familiar with *hatha yoga*, which includes a sequence of physical postures known as *asanas*. These postures place the body in positions that cultivate relaxation, concentrated awareness, and a meditative state while massaging, stretching, and stimulating the internal organs. Asanas also open and clear the energy channels and chakras within the mind and body.

Some of the forms of yoga we will cover in this book include rhythmic breathing exercises called *pranayama* and rhythmic chanting of sacred sounds known as *mantras*. Pranayama clears the energy passageways in the body and charges the chakras. Mantra practice calms and brings the mind into a one-pointed state of awareness. We will also learn *mudras*, holding the hands or body in precise positions that create specific energy circuits within the body, and *bandhas*, muscular locks that prevent the loss of *prana*, or the life force, from the body. Performing the physical asanas purifies, strengthens, and prepares the body for these practices. Therefore, it is highly recommended that you practice the asanas in conjunction with the techniques included in this program.

Nada Yoga

Nada yoga, another yogic discipline, evolved from the study of the influence of rhythm and tuning on consciousness. The primary concept of nada yoga is that ultimate reality emanates from a primordial first sound, the pulse or big bang that creates the universe. The frequencies of this root vibration create our physical world. As human beings, we are also emanations of this vibration and subject to the laws of sound.

This archetypal pulse of consciousness vibrates within us as the sound of our own heart beating. The mind and body throb to this constant rhythm of the life force. In nada yoga, the practitioner seeks communion with this pulsing vibration behind all sound—known as the *bindu*, the compacted unmanifested point beyond space and time from which creation springs. The bindu is the heartbeat behind all heartbeats.

The sound of the drum has represented this primordial pulse of creation since the beginning of human ritual. All drumming echoes this cosmic beat along with the first sound we hear in the womb—the pulse of our mother's blood. Our consciousness took physical form to this sound. This powerful pulse draws us back to our earliest stirrings of awareness and is why drumming has been used in shamanistic, religious, and transformative rites since Paleolithic times. The power of rhythmic sound returns us to the pre-socialized and unconditioned state of awareness we experienced in the womb. The seventh track on the enclosed CD is the guided Purification of the Chakras Meditation. It has been specifically designed to maximize the transformative effects of chanting mantras to the primordial rhythms of the drum.

Mantras

The rhythmic repetition of sacred sounds in the form of mantras energizes and transforms the vibrational level of the body, brain, and nervous system. Mantras are written in *Sanskrit*, the religious script of India and one of the roots of Indo-European languages. It is an old and universal thought that the light of the Divine takes the form of sacred letters and then speaks through the power of holy words.

According to Hindu tradition, the fifty seed sounds of the Sanskrit alphabet pulse from the cosmic drum of *Shiva*, the ancient god of India who drums and dances the world into being. Known as *bija mantras*, they are eternal, conscious, living sounds—serving as the root elements of speech and expressing the structure of consciousness. Through the power of words and language, we are able to think, communicate, and construct our reality.

The power of each seed sound affects the unconscious contents of the mind at the deepest levels. These bija sounds purify and dissolve the samskaras driving our behavior. Each bija mantra possesses its own particular transformative power and represents an elemental force of creation, the power of *Kundalini Shakti*. Shiva is the source of creation, the void; while Shakti is the sound of creation, the power. Shiva and Shakti embody archetypal concepts of the duality of existence, the two principles of creation, such as yin and yang, male and female, positive and negative, mental and physical.

Before creation, Shiva and Shakti are united in a matrix of undifferentiated consciousness. As the first sound occurs—the first stroke on Shiva's drum—Shakti separates from Shiva in the form of the fifty seed sounds, and creation begins. As she leaves Shiva and the seventh chakra, Shakti creates the six dimensions of reality that exist within our minds and bodies as the six chakras, in the same way that a pebble dropped into a lake creates a series of concentric circles. The sixth chakra is the realm of the most refined vibration and the nearest to the seventh chakra, or energy of Shiva. The fifth chakra is the realm of space, still very subtle but not as refined as the dimension of the sixth chakra. Kundalini Shakti continues her descent and creates the fourth chakra from the elemental energy of air, then the third chakra from fire, the second chakra from water, and finally the first and root chakra is formed of earth, the most dense and material level of reality. Here at the base chakra, she coils up and falls asleep.

Shiva as pure but formless consciousness is located at the crown of the head at the seventh chakra. Kundalini Shakti as the active, embodied power of consciousness resides in the Muladhara, or root chakra at the base of the spine. Shiva and Shakti represent the two poles of our life force. The purpose of all yogic practices is to awaken the sleeping power of Kundalini Shakti—causing a resurrection of her energy, illuminating each chakra as she returns to the source, the supreme consciousness of Shiva. This reunion results in a blissfully charged, ecstatic state, as the individual consciousness merges once again into the ultimate Self.

Prana

Pranayama breathing exercises are a primary means for awakening Kundalini. On the air rides the life force known as *prana*. This infinite and all-pervading creative energy of the universe animates the mind and body. Prana emanates from the bindu, the center and source of everything. Pranayama practices generate and store pranic energy within the chakras. The charged and stored prana can fuel self-development, healing emotional and physical imbalances.

Prana powers the physical, emotional, and mental processes that express our personality. When we have too little prana, we are subject to depression, lethargy, and irritability. We simply do not have enough energy to feel good. When prana is enhanced and accumulated, it is easier to control our reactions to circumstances and develop the powers of patience and calm awareness. People with enhanced prana are more charismatic, more influential, and more fascinating, radiating confidence and authentic power.

The Nadis

The flow of prana links the physical, mental, and spiritual dimensions of our consciousness through the structure of the chakras. The passageways of prana in the body actually create the chakras and the energy network of the mind and body. These flowing channels of energy form a system called the *nadi chakra*, the force field that surrounds each human being. This radiating field of energy is composed of thousands of *nadis*, which are very fine, wire-like currents of prana. The nadis distribute prana and consciousness to every cell in our bodies. When they are impure or blocked, the flow of prana and consciousness is disrupted. The body becomes fatigued and lethargic, and the higher thinking processes of the brain are suppressed.

While there are at least 72,000 nadis within the mind/body complex, three carry the most voltage. The primary, central pranic channel, known as the *sushumna*, travels through the spinal column, from the first chakra at the base of the spine to the sixth chakra in the center of the brain. Sushumna is the evolutionary pathway our spiritual energy must travel to reach the highest Self.

The two other subsidiary channels interweave around the sushumna from the first chakra to the sixth chakra. The left channel, *ida*, is the carrier of feminine, lunar, and mental energy. It originates at the left base of the spine and spirals upward, connecting to the left eye, left nostril, and right hemisphere of the brain, which controls the movement of the left side of the body. The right channel, *pingala*, is the carrier of masculine, active, solar, and physical energy. Pingala connects the right base of the spine to the right nostril, right eye, and left hemisphere of the brain, controlling the movement of the right side of the body.

The chakras exist as the intersections of these three major channels. Pranic energy flows through these passageways like rivers flowing through the body. The two smaller tributaries of the ida and pingala intertwine through the major river of the sushumna. When rivers merge, whirlpools or vortexes are created. When currents of energy in the body merge, circular matrixes of energy take form. These vortexes, the fusion of the physical (pingala), the mental (ida), and the spiritual (sushumna) energies, contain phenomenal possibilities of power. When cleared and charged through yogic practices, inconceivable realms of consciousness emerge within the chakras.

Bija Mantras

The chakras are symbolized by the lotus flower, the classic symbol of the womb of consciousness. Each lotus petal represents a subtle pathway of prana connecting to a chakra. Prana pulses through these power points, animating the mind and body and generating a specific humming vibration. The sound created when the chakra is balanced and flowing is recognized as one of the bija seed mantras. The chanting of the seed syllable will help tune, balance, and restore the chakra to a luminous state.

The seed mantra is also the sound of the elemental energy of the chakra. The first chakra embodies the energy of the earth element, and its seed sound is *Lang. Vang* is the sound of water at the second chakra. *Rang* is fire at the third chakra. *Yang* is air at the fourth chakra, and *Hang* is the sound of space at the fifth chakra. *Aum* embodies the sound of illuminated consciousness at the sixth chakra. The seventh chakra is the realm of the purest and most subtle awareness. The 1,000 petals of this chakra's lotus contain all fifty seed syllables of the Sanskrit alphabet, the body of Kundalini Shakti, repeated twenty times.

Yantras

Each lotus contains symbols representing the energies within the chakra, creating a geometric diagram known as a *yantra*. This is an instructional map of the charged power and consciousness in the chakra, and the yantra functions to center and draw attention inward for meditation.

The underlying layers of material reality are molecular structures in geometric patterns. Our consciousness, at the abstract symbolic level, reflects this deepest plane of reality. The yantras are actually visions of the archetypal structures of the mind revealed in geometric symbols. Concentration on the yantra awakens and loosens the samskaras in the unconscious mind. Reveries, visions, dreams, and meditations stirred by the yantra illuminate and dissolve these blockages. By meditating on the yantra, we create a field of power in the mind that clears the samskaras with minimal emotional turbulence. A brief glimpse at a yantra will have little to no impact. It takes sustained and concentrated periods of meditation on a yantra for it to imprint and transform the mind.

A small dot in the center of the yantra represents the bindu, the center of reality—the center of our true Self. The bindu represents the union of Shiva and Shakti. Beyond space and time, it is the primal Self from which the entire universe springs.

The chanting of mantras is enhanced with visual concentration on a yantra and reflects an ancient awareness of how our brain functions. The brain is divided into two hemispheres that are basically split in their control of the thinking process. The right brain functions as the creative, visual, and emotional center. The left brain is the rational, analytical, and verbal administrator.

Hemispheric Synchronization, or the Awakened Mind

Generally, either the right or left brain dominates in cycles lasting from thirty minutes to three hours. While one hemisphere is dominant, the memories, skills, and information of the other hemisphere are far less available, residing in a subconscious realm. But in states of intense creativity, deep meditation, or under the influence of rhythmic sound, both hemispheres may become entrained and function simultaneously. This state of unified whole brain functioning is called *hemispheric synchronization*, or the awakened mind.

In a state of hemispheric synchronization, we draw on both the left and the right hemispheres at the same time. The mind becomes sharper, more lucid, synthesizing information much more rapidly than normal. Emotions are easier to understand and transform. The conscious and unconscious levels of the mind communicate and integrate more easily. Insight quickens and creative intuition flourishes, giving us the ability to visualize and manifest ideas quickly. Scientists believe that hemispheric synchronization may be the neurological basis of transcendent states of consciousness.

Many religious practices seem to have originated in attempts to induce these mystical experiences. Chanting rhythmically while gazing at geometric figures—as with the combination of mantra and yantra—simultaneously engages the verbal skills of the left brain and the visual skills of right brain. Many traditional yogic practices appear to be effective techniques for synchronizing both hemispheres of the brain.

Kundalini Shakti

In the average person, the chakras normally operate at only a small percentage of their full capacity. As we clear the nadis of obstructions through yogic practices, more energy flows through them, causing the lotuses to flower more powerfully, generating radiant physical health and vitality. As the chakras become energized, their beneficial qualities become activated within our personality. Pranic energy floods the inactive, sleeping regions of the mind, transforming and refining the personality.

Kundalini Shakti, the primordial energy that can awaken the chakras, lies sleeping at the base of the spine in the form of the life force. To return our consciousness to the crown chakra and ultimate awareness, she must be awakened. The *Sat-Cakra-Nirupana*, a classical yogic text, describes the awakened Kundalini: "She is beautiful like a chain of lightning and fine like a lotus fiber, and shines in the minds of the sages. She is extremely subtle; the awakener of pure knowledge; the embodiment of all bliss, whose true nature is pure consciousness. She is symbolized as a downward pointing triangle radiating the light of ten million suns and is creation, existence, and dissolution, the power behind creation."[2]

When the energy of Kundalini is aroused through yoga practices, she surges up the spine in a coiling wave of fire, heat, and light, opening the six chakras. She rises from the Muladhara chakra as the earth energy, dissolving into water energy as she enters the second chakra. Reaching the third chakra, the water evaporates into fire. As she ascends to the fourth chakra, fire dissipates into air, and at the fifth chakra, air is absorbed into space. As she arrives at the sixth chakra, space is absorbed into the primordial energy of meditative awareness. At the crown chakra, she fuses with Shiva in a transcendental union of cosmic forces. When Kundalini rises, the chakras illuminate, activating vast areas of the brain that normally lie dormant, awakening the mind into a supreme state of Realization. The mind, an aspect of the eternal awareness embodied within the seventh chakra, contains the totality of the awakened dimensions of consciousness of the six lower chakras. This is the true nature and potential of the mind.

Awakening Kundalini and returning to full consciousness is not easy. It requires a process of disciplined practice, and authentic teachers. The chakras have to be opened and activated, and the sushumna must be cleared of obstructions. These psychological barriers within our unconscious block the complete expression of our true Self and often manifest as the very challenges that cause us to abandon our yoga practice. If yoga is pursued in a systematic and determined manner, detachment develops, and we stop identifying with the shifting waves of emotions continually arising in our minds. We become less imprisoned by past habits and begin to recognize our true identity beyond all personal psychological states. The ultimate Self begins to shine through our minds and bodies. ❁

CHAPTER
THREE

The Sixth Chakra

Command Central: Power of Awareness

WE BEGIN OUR EXPLORATION of the individual chakras with the sixth chakra, Ajna, the most evolved dimension of consciousness within the mind and body. It may seem unusual to begin our discussion with the sixth chakra, but there is a very good reason to do this—with our mind grounded in Ajna, we can safely awaken the lower chakras. Each chakra contains a storehouse of samskaras, the effects of past actions and habitual behaviors. These samskaras are both positive and negative, painful and pleasant, and hold varying degrees of emotional intensity. Due to blockages in our awareness, we are not conscious of much of this material although it continually affects our behavior. As we energize and balance each chakra, the unconscious blockages are released, and information floods into our conscious awareness. Unconscious material suddenly released into the conscious mind, without a stabilizing context to process it, can jolt the structure of our personality. If we have anchored our awareness in the higher dimensions of the sixth chakra first, we are better able to cope with this process. Many of the practices in this program will stabilize awareness at Ajna, allowing us to balance and energize the other chakras safely.

The yantra of Ajna chakra is a lotus with two brilliantly shining luminescent petals, representing the two hemispheres of the brain (see color plate "Sixth Chakra"). This double radiation of power symbolizes the energy of the moon traveling through ida nadi and connecting to the right hemisphere of the brain, and the energy of the sun traveling through pingala nadi and connecting to the left hemisphere. Within the two-petaled lotus shines the crystalline, pure white circle symbolizing the void that is the source of what is known as "All That Is." This is the original cloud of undifferentiated, unmanifested energy—the element of primordial mind. Within the circle is a downward-pointing triangle representing the seat of the supreme creative power of Kundalini Shakti. The triangle shines like the brilliant rays of the midday sun, and is heard as the primordial seed syllable, Aum, the sound of creation.

Aum, the sound of the past, the present, and the future occurring simultaneously, resembles the buzzing of bees. It is heard at Ajna chakra, where the three main nadis—ida, pingala, and sushumna—unite in the center of the brain. These three channels originate in the Muladhara chakra at the base of the spine. Ida spirals upward to the left through the chakras, coming to the top of the spine, meeting pingala and sushumna in the sixth chakra, and continues to the left nostril, influencing the right brain. Pingala spirals upwards to the right through the chakras, coming to the top of the spine to join pingala and sushumna in the sixth chakra, and continues to the right nostril, influencing the left brain. Sushumna runs directly up from the Muladhara to the Ajna chakra. The intersection of these three pranic forces in Ajna chakra creates the buzzing sound of Aum. When Ajna is fully activated, sushumna will continue its flow up to the crown chakra.

The sixth chakra is the highest junction of these three power lines. Pingala is prana, the life force; and ida is *chitta*, consciousness and knowing. Pingala is the physical energy of the body; ida is mental energy; and sushumna is the flow of spiritual energy. The sushumna opens as the result of the balanced interaction between ida and pingala—mind and body—giving rise to the spiritual force in our lives. At Ajna chakra, the body, mind, and spirit fuse into the ultimate manifestation of our human consciousness.

As awareness becomes concentrated and purified at the merging of these three great forces, the individual sense of ego fades. Within the lower chakras, ego awareness is always present and functions as the background for all experiences. It is not until ida and pingala unite with sushumna in Ajna chakra that the ego dissolves as the filter for awareness.

Called the "Eye of Knowledge," Ajna chakra is the seat of the cognitive mind and its intellectual, reasoning, and mental abilities. With an activated sixth chakra, intelligence, concentration, and memory expand, and the mind becomes strong and steady. The Sanskrit roots of Ajna mean "to know," and "to command." This Lotus of Command coordinates the five sense perceptions and dimensions of awareness embodied in the lower five chakras. All incoming information from the body's sense organs comes into the brain through the sixth chakra for processing. The cognitive mind functions as the sixth sense, perception—the organizing consciousness that receives information from the five sense organs. It gathers and interprets based on past experiences and belief structures. The cognitive mind is a fusion of what we have learned and what we believe—a combination of personal experiences, emotional patterns, and memories. We identify these familiar structures of thinking and emotions as our mind. And through our sense perceptions and memory, we create our perception of reality.

There are specific meditation practices to purify the consciousness that interprets the sense perceptions, so that we begin to perceive the world directly, rather than through our belief systems. *Trataka*, staring at a candle flame while cutting all thoughts, allows the mind to simply and directly perceive light. Following the breath and focusing all awareness on the sensations of inhaling and exhaling while cutting attachment to our thoughts is a traditional purification of the sense perception of feeling. Repetition of sounds in mantra practice is another way of suspending thoughts and concentrating on sound perception without attaching meaning to it.

These practices develop the witnessing aspect of our mind so that we become detached observers not only of events but also of our own thoughts. As awareness develops, we begin to see the hidden structure underlying visible appearances. When the witnessing aspect of Ajna awakens, the meaning and significance of symbols flashes into our conscious mind. Our intuition flowers, and extrasensory perception arises. We perceive the reality of the moment rather than our habitual thoughts about reality. Our choices become congruent with what is actually occurring, and we learn to live fully in the present moment.

Our ego attachments determine how long we stay at each level of awareness, or chakra. The forces at the first chakra represent inertia. As long as our material needs are being met—food, shelter, and security—we are content to remain there, with no desire to change or expand into any other state of awareness. To transcend the earth element is to gather the energy to begin the expansion of consciousness. At the second chakra, we realize we cannot find our self only in relationship to others, but must develop our relationship to our self. At the third chakra, we find out that owning, conquering, and controlling everything does not lead to contentment or happiness. At the fourth chakra, we realize the universal power of love. Here we experience the joy of giving, caring, and nurturing ourselves and others with love and kindness. At the fifth chakra, we begin to understand that the outer world is a projection of our own inner reality, giving rise to a sense of detachment which releases us into higher states of awareness. Evolving into the sixth chakra, we move into the non-dual state of realizing there is only One of us here, and there is only the present moment.

Yantra Meditation Instructions for the Sixth Chakra

The Ajna chakra is visually represented by a geometric power diagram known as a yantra, a meditation tool that awakens the hidden structure of the dimensions of consciousness contained within the chakra. The traditional meaning of *yantra* is "loom," "instrument," or "machine," and it is used to transform the personality by drawing your attention into the core of your consciousness. As you gaze at the yantra, attention is drawn into the center to focus on the black dot called the *bindu*, which represents the center of all things, the center of the self, the center of ultimate consciousness. The yantra is a means of introducing your mind to its infinite source.

• It is ideal to place the Ajna yantra (see color plate "Sixth Chakra") at reading distance, with the bindu in the center of the yantra at eye level. You can prop the book open in any way where the page remains flat (I use a music stand), and you can cover the facing page with a blank sheet of paper.

• This yantra is a lotus with two white petals containing a translucent full moon. Within the full moon is a pale yellow triangle with a bright white flame in its center.

• Take a seated posture with the spine straight.

- Gaze with a soft focus at the center of the yantra. Do not move the eyes around, looking at different aspects of the diagram, but keep your eyes focused on the bindu so that you can see the entire yantra.
- Practice the Full Yogic Breath along with Track One on the enclosed CD, after reading the instructions for this practice given on page 64. As you do the breathing practice, let your consciousness be drawn into the bindu.

LISTEN TO TRACK 1
Full Yogic Breath

- The Full Yogic Breath track on the CD is five minutes long, which is the ideal amount of time to do this practice. Commit to completing the entire five minutes. Eventually you should practice without using the CD, and it is ideal to set a timer so that you do not need to glance away to check the time. With a timer or alarm set, you can let all thoughts subside, keeping the soft focus on the yantra and the awareness on your breath. It is perfectly fine to extend the duration of the meditation on the yantra. ✺

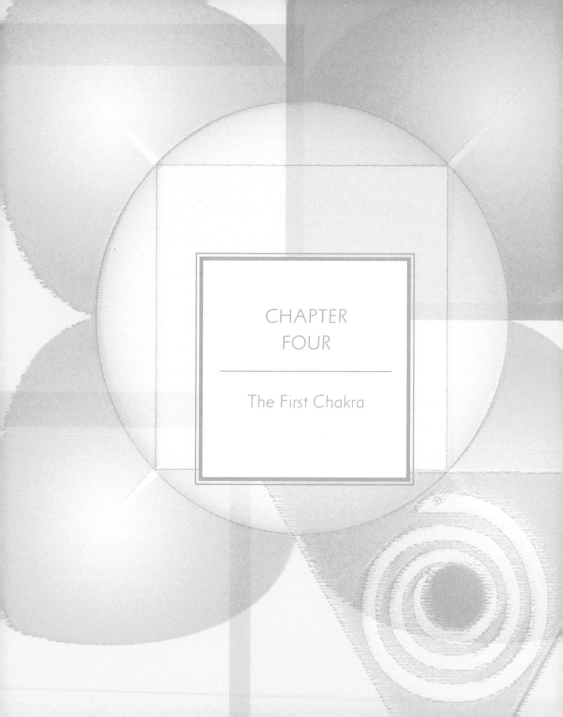

CHAPTER
FOUR

The First Chakra

The Root Support: Tribal Power

THE FIRST CHAKRA, the Muladhara chakra, is located just below the base of the spine at the perineum. In Sanskrit, *mula* means "root," and *adhara* translates as "the support." *Adhara* also means "perineum." The Muladhara—the foundation of the energy structure of human consciousness—is the support of all the other chakras.

The earth element of Muladhara represents the quality of solidity, gravity, and weight. This is the root center of physical experience. The instinctive fears surrounding physical survival, abandonment by the group, loss of home, family, and social order originate at this chakra. The primary drive is for security and comfort.

First chakra issues that bind us are social indoctrination, concepts of law and order, family and social honor codes, and feelings of obligated support and loyalty. We worry not only about ourselves but also about our family, friends, and the groups we identify with.

The forces that keep us from changing are strong here. "Just leave well enough alone," and "Don't rock the boat," could be the mantras of this chakra. "Don't risk what you have for something outside of the box" is thinking straight out of Muladhara. We feel compelled to fit in and be normal. Worry and anxiety are instinctive responses to first chakra issues. The goal of yoga is to release and transcend these debilitating emotions, allowing us to see our lives from a higher vantage point.

The yantra of the Muladhara chakra is a deep red, four-petaled lotus representing the four directions (see color plate "First Chakra"). Within the lotus is a yellow square symbolizing the elemental energy of earth. In the center of the yellow square is a red triangle that expresses the creative energy of Kundalini Shakti. Inside the triangle is a *lingam*, traditionally a symbol of a phallus, with a red serpent, the sleeping Kundalini, coiled around it three and one half times. Kundalini is the cosmic manifestation of prana, the life force, in the individual body. She is the entire cosmic experience from creation to dissolution.

The three coils of the sleeping Kundalini represent the form of the mantra Aum. This primordial seed sound symbolizes the triadic nature of existence, including our conscious, subconscious, and unconscious; our waking, dreaming, and deep sleep states; and the past, present, and future. The half coil represents the fourth, transcendental nature of reality. When Kundalini sleeps, her head blocks the opening of the sushumna, the main energy channel in the center of the spine. Traditionally, the sushumna is visualized as a silvery tube running from the first chakra to the sixth chakra. When properly aroused, Kundalini Shakti streams upward through sushumna into the crown chakra, the Sahasrara. She is endless time, the eternal goddess of the beginning and ending of life. In most people, she lies sleeping in the womb of the unconscious. In her dormant state, she is that instinctive level of life that supports our basic existence. When she begins to awaken, she represents our spiritual potential. Both of these possibilities lie in Muladhara. We may go through life conscious or unconscious.

The *kanda* is the origin of the thousands of nadis, or energy meridians of the subtle body, and is located in the Muladhara. This bulb-shaped energy complex, about three inches wide by nine inches long, extends from the Muladhara up into the Manipura chakra at the navel. The yogic *mula bandha* practice, the rhythmic contracting of the muscles in the area of the perineum, squeezes and stimulates the kanda, pulsing energy up the spine and throughout the nadis. The three major nadis—the ida, pingala, and sushumna—originate together in the kanda and meet at the top of the spine at the sixth chakra.

Psychic knots, complexes of intertangled energy and consciousness, block sushumna at different points, and must be unraveled for Kundalini to move to a higher state of consciousness. In the Muladhara, the identification of our consciousness with the physical body and our sense perceptions produces what is known as "the Knot of Creation," or our misconception that the material world is all there is. Muladhara represents the level of physical creation. Nothing seems more real to the average person than the earthbound, sensual, and material attachments of the Muladhara chakra. The elemental energy of earth is that which is solid, resistant, and stable within ourselves. Muladhara connects us to the earth through the force of gravity, the power that holds things together from the molecular level of atomic particles to the cosmic level of the solar system and the galaxies. At this chakra, we find ourselves rooted in the actual feelings of our bodies; nothing seems more immediately real than our bodies and how they exist within gravity.

No sense perception is more primordially identified with bodily experience than the power of smell, the sense perception of the first chakra. Scents penetrate to the deepest levels of the unconscious mind, either attracting us toward something enticing or repulsing us from disagreeable and possibly dangerous odors. It is the oldest sense perception and has a more direct pathway to the brain and nervous system than any of the other five senses. The olfactory nerves activated by the chemical messengers of fragrance directly stimulate the brain and the pituitary gland, which controls the human hormonal system. Researchers have shown that odors can instantaneously change a person's state of consciousness. The olfactory bulb in the brain extends back from the eyebrow center, the trigger point for Ajna chakra in the center of the brain. Pranayama breathing practices and specific smells effectively stimulate this link between Muladhara and Ajna chakras. Whatever affects either of these chakras immediately affects the other; they are the two opposite ends of the sushumna.

The work organ is the anus, with its function of releasing what is processed and no longer needed in the body. On a physical level, healthy elimination is essential to our well-being. And on the subtle psychological and emotional level, releasing negative patterns of behavior and thinking clears many issues blocking the chakras.

Developing the power to do this begins in the Muladhara when we start releasing our attachment to first chakra fears. These fears are instinctive; we will always have them, yet we do not have to allow them unconscious control over our decisions. We can release our fears by allowing them to come fully into consciousness, properly evaluating their validity and then allowing them to subside.

The animal power of this chakra, the elephant, progresses calmly, alertly, and skillfully through life. This powerful, grounded animal embodies the stability and solidity of the earth. The elephant symbolizes the potent yet dormant power of Kundalini Shakti residing in a stationary, secure, and enduring place.

The bija syllable that represents the overall frequency of this chakra is Lang, the seed sound of the elemental energy of earth. It is the sound of the nourishing and sustaining energy of the earth. The quality of the earth element on the physical level is represented by the flesh and bones of the body, and symbolizes the mind's ability to serve as the ground for all experience. Chanting Lang energizes and rebalances the first chakra. As Muladhara comes into balance, first chakra insecurities and anxieties give way to inner strength and a strong sense of unwavering security.

Muladhara, the first chakra at the base of the spine, and Ajna, the sixth chakra at the top of the spine in the center of the brain, are the two powerful end poles of the major energy channel running through the body. The flow of energy originates at Muladhara and functions as the direct switch for awakening Ajna. Pranic energy is generated at Muladhara; stored in Manipura, the navel chakra; purified at Vishuddha, the throat chakra; and distributed from Ajna chakra throughout the energetic structure of the mind and body. At the first chakra, Kundalini is the Shakti of physical manifestation. At the Ajna chakra, she is the Shakti of the mental and psychic realm; and at the crown chakra, she is the Shakti of the spiritual realm. When Kundalini sleeps, we are awake to this world. When she is awakened, we lose consciousness of the world, and our attention passes into the realm of formless or infinite consciousness.

To become truly conscious demands a tremendous amount of energy, strength, and endurance. This is why we cannot leave it to the end of our life. At that point, we will not have the energy or time to become awakened. We can begin now by becoming aware of our thoughts, move into evaluating our beliefs, and then we can choose to dissolve those that stand in the way of our spiritual growth. This kind of personal transformation often separates us from our family and community.

The tribal mind is the power of sharing a belief system with other members. We are connected through our first chakra to our family and our cultural tribal mind. We begin to transcend the first chakra by freeing ourselves from the constant struggle to meet our family's and friends' expectations and from the tyranny of societal obligations. We begin consciously letting go of limitations and internal conflicts, clearing the channels for the next stage of growth. Muladhara is the place of the beginning, the gateway to the spiritual path.

Yantra Meditation Instructions for the First Chakra

- It is ideal to place the Muladhara yantra (see color plate "First Chakra") at reading distance with the bindu in the center of the yantra at eye level. You can prop the book open in any way where the page remains flat (I use a music stand), and you can cover the facing page with a blank sheet of paper.
- This yantra is a deep red four-petaled lotus. In the center of the lotus is a bright yellow square containing a beautiful bright red triangle shining like the rising sun. The triangle is pointing downward. Inside the triangle is the bindu point of ultimate consciousness. Coiled around this bindu is kundalini shakti, the source of our life force, her body an electric coil of the lightning-like energy of prana.
- Take a seated posture with the spine straight.
- Gaze with a soft focus at the center of the yantra. Do not move the eyes around looking at different aspects of the diagram, but keep your eyes focused on the bindu so that you can see the entire yantra.
- Practice the Full Yogic Breath along with Track One on the enclosed CD after reading the instructions for this practice given on page 64. As you do the breathing practice, let your consciousness be drawn into the bindu.

LISTEN TO TRACK 1
Full Yogic Breath

- The Full Yogic Breath track on the CD is five minutes long, which is the ideal amount of time to do this practice. Commit to completing the entire five minutes. Eventually you should practice without using the CD, and it is ideal to set a timer so that you do not need to glance away to check the time. With a timer or alarm set, you can let all thoughts subside, keeping the soft focus on the yantra and the awareness on your breath. It is perfectly fine to extend the duration of the meditation on the yantra. ☀

CHAPTER
FIVE

The Second Chakra

The Seat of the Self: Power of Relationships

IN 1932, Carl Jung held a special conference on the study of Kundalini Yoga, describing the journey through the chakras as a method of psychic hygiene. This marked a milestone in the psychological understanding of Eastern systems of personal transformation. Viewing the structure of the chakras as a model for the evolutionary stages of higher consciousness, he described the Muladhara as the earth realm where Kundalini sleeps and most people go about their lives instinctually and unconsciously. When Kundalini begins to stir and awareness moves up to the second chakra, the journey into the symbolic depths of the unconscious begins: "The very first demand of a mystery cult always has been to go into water, into the baptismal fount. The way into any higher development leads through water, with the danger of being swallowed by the monster" (the *makara*, a mythological crocodile).[3] He spoke of the second chakra as "the mandala of baptism, or of rebirth, or of destruction—whatever the consequence of the baptism may be."[4] For Jung, the early Christian rite of baptism was a symbolic drowning, from which a newborn person emerged.

Svadisthana, the second chakra, is located in the lower abdomen, very near and tightly interwoven with the energy of the first chakra. The yantra of the second chakra is a white crescent moon within a circle, in the center of a six-petaled vermilion lotus, symbolizing the element of water ruled by the moon (see color plate "Second

Chakra"). Water represents the continuity, adaptability, and flowing quality of the mind and the blood in the body. The sense perception connected to Svadisthana and water is taste.

Vang is the bija syllable for the frequency of water and the energy of the second chakra. Chanting Vang balances the energy of the second chakra and refines our sense of taste literally and metaphorically, giving rise to insight, refinement, discrimination, and wisdom in all areas of creative thought.

Desire rules this chakra, and the leading desires are focused on sexuality, relationships, and procreation. Inspiration to create starts in the second chakra and can develop as the drive to bring new life into being. It also manifests as the urge to give birth to our dreams; people who are dominated by second chakra energy often become artists, poets, musicians, or dancers.

Svadisthana chakra acts as the activating switch to the unconscious mind and its collection of samskaras, the unconscious imprints that are the background of our personality. The dimensions of this chakra hold our karma, our past lives, and the imprints of our experiences in this life. These impressions shape our consciousness, profoundly affecting our emotions and behavior. In discussing the second chakra as the repository of the unconscious, Swami Satyananda Saraswati, the founder of the Bihar School of Yoga in India, said, "Svadisthana is made up of all the rubbish which you never wanted, which you never needed, which you never desired but which got in."[5]

Svadisthana means "the dwelling place of the Self," or "one's own abode," and is the seat of our unconscious behavior. Who we are unconsciously is really the projection of our samskaras. The drives of the second chakra seem to function autonomously, overriding other aspects of our intelligence and the conscious mind, particularly when it comes to food and sex. Baptism into the second chakra is a plunge into the depths of the unconscious. We surface anointed with a dawning awareness of the subconscious factors driving our behavior.

The makara, a crocodile creature, is the animal power of this chakra. Metaphorically floating on the surface of the mind, eyes above in the conscious world, body hidden under the water in the unconscious, the makara can snap and devour suddenly, pulling its unsuspecting prey under the surface of the water. This mythic crocodile also represents an aspect of the structure of our brain. Influential 20th century scientist

Carl Sagan described this in his book, Cosmos, "According to a provocative insight by Paul MacLean, the higher functions of the brain evolved in three successive stages. Capping the brain stem is the R-complex, the seat of aggression, ritual, territoriality, and social hierarchy, which evolved hundreds of millions of years ago in our reptilian ancestors. Deep inside the skull of every one of us, there is something like the brain of a crocodile."[6] This is the lower brain, the seat of the subconscious. Our fear of being swallowed by the makara is really the fear of being overcome by our subconscious issues.

Intimately connected with the first and second chakras, the reptilian brain is focused on ensuring survival and maintaining physical well-being, hoarding, dominance, mating, and preening. The reptilian complex is heavily influenced by rhythm, and is rebalanced and soothed by rhythmic movement, sound, or routines. This is why regular periods of meditation, yoga, and rhythmic practices such as pranayama and mantra are very effective tools for refining consciousness.

Directly affected by sound, our emotions and consciousness can be reorganized and purified by chanting bija mantras while gazing at the yantra of the chakra. Each bija sound affects the unconscious contents at the deepest levels of the mind, while the geometric structure visually vibrates our consciousness. This practice purges the unconscious mind of the samskaras blocking awareness and the flow of prana through the mind and body.

In Muladhara, the goal is for financial security, and as the person evolves into the second chakra, the focus of attention is drawn toward sensual desires and fantasies. Those captivated by this energy often see themselves as princes, lords, heroes, queens, or Amazons. They may do this through creative fantasizing or by consuming TV, movies, or novels. Mythology, storytelling, and daydreaming all have their roots in this chakra, and every culture produces the legend of the destroyer of evil, the invincible hero or heroine. Hollywood is an industry based on second chakra archetypes and fascination with romantic and sexual relationships.

When attention is primarily focused at the second chakra, we seek pleasure through the tongue, the mouth, and the genital organs. We look for fulfillment through the enjoyment of food, drink, and sexuality. It is easy to stay occupied with seeking and enjoying physical pleasures and entertaining ourselves with fantasies, particularly if these were learned responses to abuse or an unhappy home life. Wounds from past relationships are stored in this chakra, and often unresolved issues from sexual and physical abuse manifest in uncontrollable desires for food, sex, or sleep.

Sexual energy is connected mainly to Svadisthana chakra, but also to the first and third chakras. When sexual energy is not satisfied or transformed into energy for other uses, if it is neglected or conditioned by abuse, then it can be expressed through Muladhara as neurotic craving for possessions or the desire for dominance and power at Manipura. To remain healthy and balanced, we must recognize and respect the natural limitations of the body and mind. Obtaining a harmonious peaceful state involves a balancing of our eating, sleeping, and sexual behaviors.

Our relationships reflect our unconscious choices and motivations, and also our relationship to ourselves. Each relationship can serve as a mirror, helping us to see our less-than-conscious selves more clearly, and understand our conditioning. Our culture hammers into us the idea that we are only valued in relationships. Women in particular are taught that their value is determined by whom they can attract. Magazines, TV, and radio commercials continually broadcast the message that women must constantly improve their physical appearance to accomplish this goal. To individuate into an autonomous person valuing oneself beyond relationships is nearly impossible.

We are tied to the mythology of the soul mate, the one who will complete us and give meaning and joy to our lives. Master yogi Baba Hari Dass, when asked about the concept of soul mates, stated, "The soul does not mate. The samskaras mate."[7] The soul mate we yearn for is not another person; it is the source of creation, the source of our own Self. We are the yin striving to unite with the yang. We are Shakti striving to return to Shiva. The yearning is for union with the supreme source of sacred consciousness.

The absorption we can experience with sexual relationships is also dominated by the rhythms of our hormones, rhythms that change over the course of our lives. Our hormones drive us to want to have sex. This drive is such a potent force and the consequences—reproduction—are of such magnitude, particularly for women, that all cultures have created elaborate rituals and mythologies around mating. While we are young and the hormonal drive to reproduce is strongest, we are most susceptible to our culture's mating mythologies. As we grow older and our hormonal patterns shift, we find it easier to understand what was driving us in the earlier periods of our lives. Midlife has traditionally been the time when human beings have switched their focus from social and family obligations to the pursuit of spiritual transformation.

How we experience our lives, understand ourselves and our goals, and how we proceed to fulfill them depends on the internal state of our consciousness. By balancing the energy of the second chakra, we awaken further dimensions of creativity and energy, leading to the release of the psychic knots binding Kundalini. As she awakens in a spiraling buzz of ascending consciousness, the lotuses bloom into their full power and potentialities, propelling us into ever-higher dimensions of awareness.

Yantra Meditation Instructions for the Second Chakra

- It is ideal to place the Svadisthana yantra (see color plate "Second Chakra") at reading distance with the bindu in the center of the yantra at eye level. You can prop the book open in any way where the page remains flat (I use a music stand), and you can cover the facing page with a blank sheet of paper.
- This yantra is a reddish-gold, vermilion, six-petaled lotus. In the center of the lotus is a blue circle representing the energy of the water element. Within the circle is the luminescent crescent moon.
- Take a seated posture with the spine straight.
- Gaze with a soft focus at the center of the yantra. Do not move the eyes around looking at different aspects of the diagram, but keep your eyes focused on the bindu so that you can see the entire yantra.
- Practice the Full Yogic Breath along with Track One on the enclosed CD after reading the instructions for this practice given on page 64. As you do the breathing practice, let your consciousness be drawn into the bindu.

LISTEN TO TRACK 1
Full Yogic Breath

- The Full Yogic Breath track on the CD is five minutes long, which is the ideal amount of time to do this practice. Commit to completing the entire five minutes. Eventually you should practice without using the CD, and it is ideal to set a timer so that you do not need to glance away to check the time. With a timer or alarm set, you can let all thoughts subside, keeping the soft focus on the yantra and the awareness on your breath. It is perfectly fine to extend the duration of the meditation on the yantra. ✸

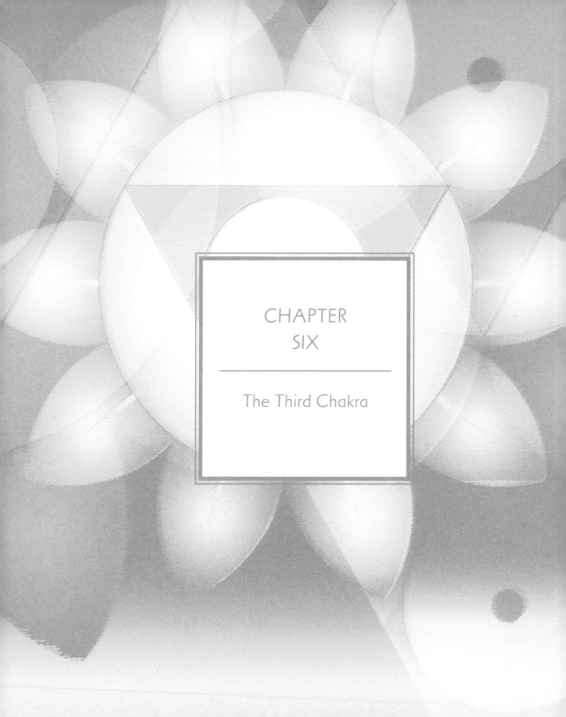

CHAPTER
SIX

The Third Chakra

The Jewel at the Navel of Reality: Personal Power

THE JOURNEY THROUGH the chakras is an initiation into conscious aware-ness. Jung describes the process as, "how consciousness came to pass, how it rises from level to level. Those were chakras, new worlds of consciousness of natural growths, one above the other. This is the symbolism of all initiation cults: the awakening out of Muladhara, and the going into the water, the baptismal fount with the danger of the makara—the devouring quality, or attribute of the sea."8 We plunged into the unconscious to be cleansed. As we free ourselves of the second chakra obstacles, we are lifted into the energy of the third chakra, Manipura, the fiery center, the place where the rising sun first appears after the baptism. The third chakra is the core of our constructed personality and ego projected out into the world. Manipura is where we become the ruling god of our own world.

Manipura means "the jeweled city." This chakra is also called *Mani Padma*, the jew-eled lotus, and the *Nabhi Padma*, the navel lotus. It is the jewel in the lotus at the navel of reality, a widespread concept in the ancient world representing the sacred stone, the *omphalos* (navel) at the base of what is known as the Tree of Life. Many temples had an omphalos stone that marked the site as a center where different dimensions of sacred energy met. For the Tree of Life, it is the place where the roots go down into the earth, the source of its nourishing, sustaining energy. For humans, the navel is the place where we were attached to the umbilical cord, the channel through which the life force, the prana, flowed into us from our mother. Our spine, our Tree of Life, our entire being grew out of this connection.

Manipura, at the solar plexus, is the center of gravity and the storehouse of pranic energy in the body. It is the brain of the digestive process, where the essence of food is extracted, digested, and transformed into energy. The energy generated at Manipura regulates and fuels the biological processes of our minds and bodies. It influences the body temperature, the small intestines, liver, spleen, stomach, pancreas, and diaphragm, and governs the adrenal glands. When this pranic energy is low, we feel lifeless—lacking vitality, motivation, and commitment—and are prone to illness and depression. Without an energized Manipura chakra, it is hard to enjoy life.

The yantra of Manipura chakra is a lotus of ten petals, the color of purple-black rain clouds, representing ten dimensions of information and awareness (see color plate "Third Chakra"). Within the lotus is a flaming red triangle shining like the setting sun. The triangle symbolizes the fiery womb of the goddess, the cosmic oven, where things are created. The elemental energy of this chakra is fire, representing the luminosity and clarity of the mind and the energy in the body. The sense perception connected to Manipura is sight. The motivating desire is to develop a powerful identity in the world through achievements.

The third chakra is associated with hungers of many different kinds, literal and metaphorical. Revered mythologist Joseph Campbell noted that Manipura's function is to be "aggressive: to conquer, to consume, to turn everything into oneself."9 Rang is the overall bija syllable for the energy of fire and the third chakra. Chanting Rang increases our digestive power and the powers to absorb and assimilate not only food, but also all forms of energy. It brings emotional and physical hungers into balance, and we understand how to appropriately satisfy the different hungers we experience.

The animal power of the third chakra is the ram, symbolizing assertiveness, endurance, and indomitable energy. This strong animal charges headfirst, battering obstacles out of the way—a bit tough on both the psyche of the one pounding objects out of

FIRST CHAKRA
Chakra Sound: Lang

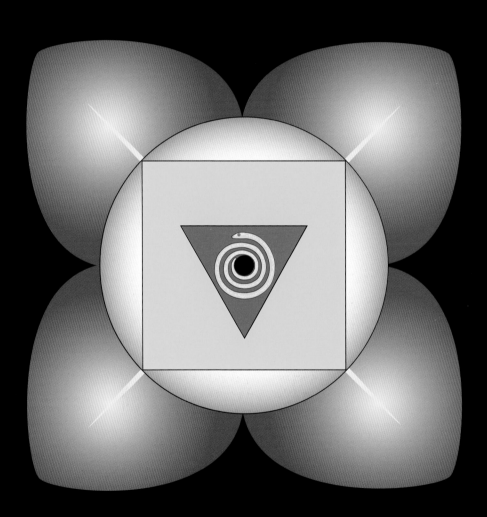

SECOND CHAKRA

Chakra Sound: Vang

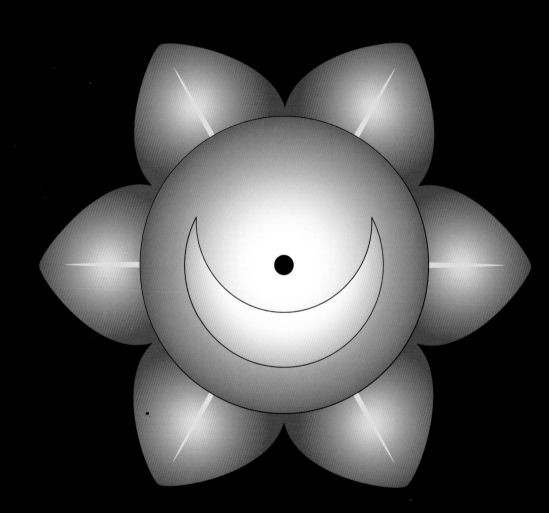

THIRD CHAKRA

Chakra Sound: Rang

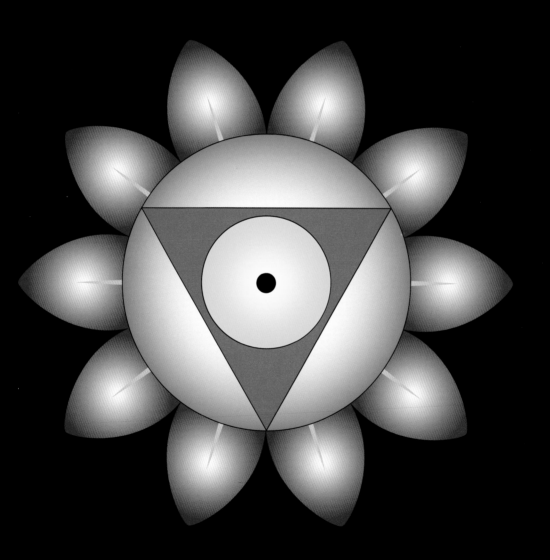

FOURTH CHAKRA

Chakra Sound: Yang

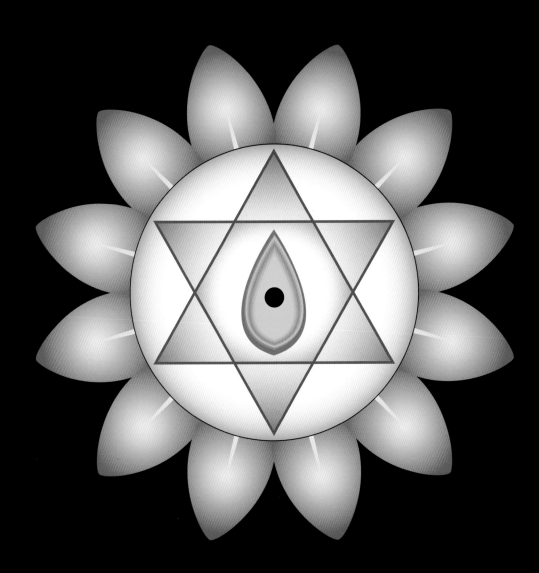

FIFTH CHAKRA
Chakra Sound: Hang

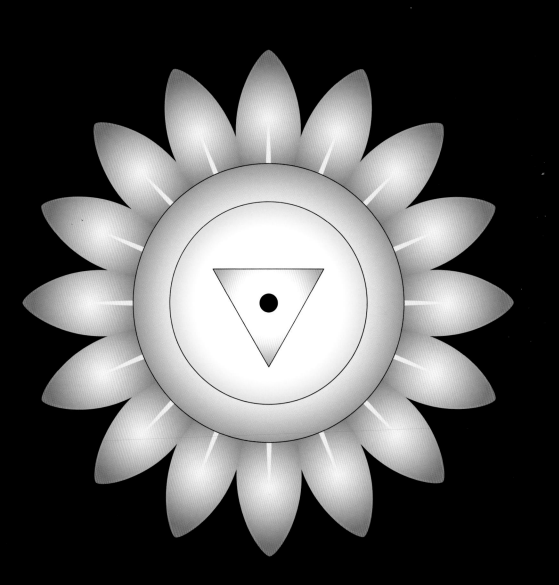

SIXTH CHAKRA

Chakra Sound: Aum

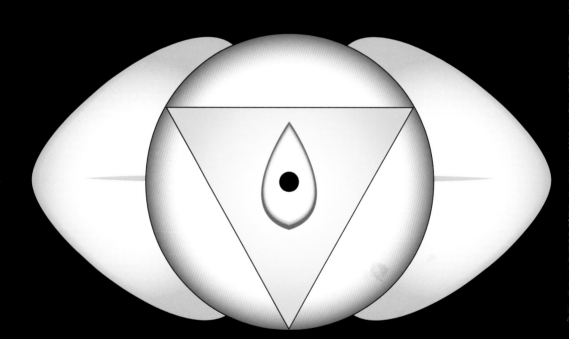

SEVENTH CHAKRA

Chakra Sound: Hangsah

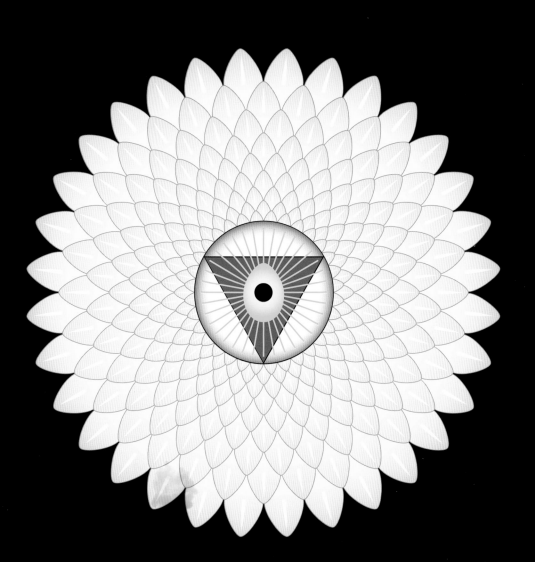

CHAKRA SYSTEM WITH THE THREE MAIN NADIS

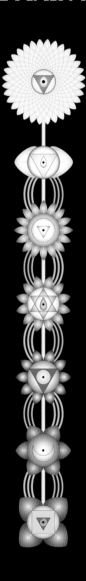

the way and the objects or people getting pounded. The ram reflects the nature of a third-chakra person, who is dominated by competitive ambition in his or her striving for recognition, immortality, and power. The sacred animal of *Agni*, the Hindu god of fire, the ram is also the astrological symbol of Aries ruled by Mars, the fiery planet of violence, rashness, impulsiveness, and vivid passions. Yet Aries also embodies the power of the life force within the vegetation that bursts through the earth in the spring.

The issues of this chakra begin to dominate during puberty, when we are compelled from within to develop our personal identity in the world. Issues of self-esteem, personal power, and how we view ourselves in the eyes of the world loom large. The first chakra functions as the staging ground of power within the tribal mind, where we create a strong sense of the self within that group mind. As we have seen, the chief issues at the first chakra are how to get our basic survival needs of food, comfort, and shelter met. The second chakra is the realm of relationships, where we explore the flow of power between the self and others, developing a strong sense of identity within the world of family and friends. At the third chakra, the field of our personal power and energetic interactions with the external world, we develop a sense of our self as an individual projecting power out into the world.

Having reached the Jeweled City at the Navel of the World, we seek our fame and fortune. We establish our own sense of authority and find our own voice. By separating from the tribal mind of the first chakra and the relationship mind of the second chakra, we free ourselves from the grasp of the group mind constantly telling us who we are. We replace the voice of the cultural mind by exploring what we believe, what we feel, what we think.

Until Manipura chakra is energized, our sense of self has been formed by the memories, experiences, emotions, and knowledge stored in the vibrational fields of the first and second chakras. In Manipura, not only is food transformed and digested, but also our concepts, our emotions, and our views of ourselves and others. To be truly self-confident with high self-esteem, we must feel secure in our world, a first chakra issue, and our relationships must be based on mutual support and respect, a second chakra issue. In the third chakra, we thoroughly question the root sources of our beliefs, recognizing them as our own and beneficial, or as detrimental and limiting beliefs inherited from our tribal mind or past experiences.

Issues we might confront in the third chakra are intimidation, anger, resentment, and fear. We may be afraid of making decisions, assuming responsibilities, or trusting those around us, but the overriding fear is of failure, rejection, criticism, and ridicule. For many people, fears rather than creative dreams rule their decisions and behavior. Countless dreams go unpursued due to these unconscious internal fears. If we do not face and constructively resolve our fears, they can activate physical and emotional illnesses that then must be addressed on the bodily level.

As Kundalini awakens and reaches this chakra, the negative potentials are transformed in the purifying fires of Manipura. The strengths of a balanced and energized third chakra include healthy self-esteem, self-respect, appropriate self-discipline, and stamina, creating an empowered sense of self. Activating this chakra lowers hypertension and ends problems of the intestinal region including indigestion, constipation, and malabsorption. We glow with vitality and can look forward to a long life—a particular goal of third chakra people.

When we set foot on our own true path, a balanced inner ambition arises. We can choose to invest in our spiritual development rather than in power over people, things, and events in the physical world. As we do this, we limit the authority of outer circumstances over our emotions, minds, and bodies, strengthening our inner spiritual Self. Replacing the influences of the social mind with inner guidance strengthens our energy field, attracting like-minded people and possibilities and warding off negative people and circumstances. We create a nurturing and sustaining network of people that support our transformation.

Aggressive and unconscious ego-centeredness dissolves, and the creativity released from balancing the second chakra now takes on a form of practicality. At Manipura chakra, visions move out of the fantasy realm and are manifested in the world. The power to command and organize develops. The ability to articulate verbally evolves along with the power to express our thoughts effectively. The traditional balancing path for this chakra is selfless service—serving the world without the desire for rewards. We gain the understanding that whatever work we do can be done as a practice of selfless service.

As we center ourselves in this chakra, our courage to take risks grows, and we are able to generate and direct actions in the world without debilitating fears and second-guessing ourselves. Our intuition evolves, becoming our own powerful, natural source of guidance. We catch fire with our own unique purpose, and we have the energy, resources, and drive to fulfill our visions.

Yantra Meditation Instructions for the Third Chakra

- It is ideal to place the Manipura yantra (see color plate "Third Chakra") at reading distance with the bindu in the center of the yantra at eye level.
- This yantra is a lotus with ten petals the color of dense purple-black rain clouds. In the center of this lotus is a red triangle representing the elemental energy of fire.
- Take a seated posture with the spine straight.
- Gaze with a soft focus at the center of the yantra. Do not move the eyes around looking at different aspects of the diagram, but keep your eyes focused on the bindu so that you can see the entire yantra.
- Practice the Full Yogic Breath along with Track One on the enclosed CD or on your own. As you do the breathing practice, let your consciousness be drawn into the bindu.

LISTEN TO TRACK 1
Full Yogic Breath

- Practice for five minutes. It is perfectly fine to extend the duration of the meditation on the yantra. ✸

CHAPTER SEVEN

The Fourth Chakra

The Unstruck Sound: Power of Compassion

THE FOURTH CHAKRA, Anahata, is located in the region of the heart. In the center of this chakra is heard the unstruck sound, the Anahata, the transcendental humming pulse of consciousness. When our thoughts dissolve and the mind merges into the energy of this chakra, we hear the buzzing, bee-like hum of the universe.

The Doctrine of Vibration from the 13th century Hindu and Buddhist culture of Kashmir describes reality as a living, pulsing field emanating from the vibration of ultimate consciousness. Each individual consciousness is a point in this luminous, rhythmic web of reality. Yet each is also the entire web, pulsing to the cosmic beat of infinite awareness. The heart chakra tells us there is only One of us here. This is the great chakra vibrating simultaneously in the hearts of all beings. As this center is energized and purified, love, faith, devotion, inspiration, and harmonious balance in our relationships unfold. Anahata's driving energy is toward unconditional compassion and lovingkindness.

Even before we are born, the first three chakras start functioning, and will be the active forces behind most peoples' lives. Many will never have goals any higher than the basic drives surrounding sex, money, power, prestige, fame, security, and comfort. And for many, these issues will revolve around sex. People seek recognition, fortune, power, possessions, beauty and bodily enhancements in order to obtain sexual partners. On these partners falls the responsibility to fulfill the rest of the lower chakras' desires: home, food, security, relationship, and love.

The issues of the first three chakras endlessly seduce, mesmerize, and fascinate us. Most therapeutic counseling focuses on these concerns. Gossip is an ancient technique for distracting ourselves by keeping the focus on first, second, and third chakra issues. Traditional spiritual teachers instruct us to bypass these chakras and take the energy directly up to the heart chakra or higher. Above the Anahata, there are three chakras concerned with spiritual evolution: Vishuddha, Ajna, and Sahasrara. The heart chakra functions as a bridge between the drives of the lower chakras and these higher chakras. At this threshold, the energy of compassion and lovingkindness draws us upward into the higher spiritual dimensions.

The elemental energy of Anahata is air, and in the air rides the life force of prana. Air is connected with the sense perception of touch, and its organ is the skin through which we feel the world. The heart center controls the circulatory, respiratory, and immune system through the connection with the physical heart, lungs, and thymus gland, the center of the body's immune system. Activation of the fourth chakra will boost the immune system to peak strength.

Our heart beats approximately seventy two times per minute, which adds up to 100,000 beats every day. Five to twenty-five quarts of blood pulse through 60,000 miles of veins, arteries, and capillaries every minute. A well-energized and balanced heart chakra has a profound influence on overall health—regulating our breathing, our heartbeat, and our circulation. Within this center, air, prana, and blood unite and keep the body and mind purified and full of vitality.

The Upanishads, sacred texts of Hinduism, say the heart is the seat of the soul, of waking consciousness and the seat of prana, the breath of life. According to the Upanishads, the *Atman*—the eternal, transcendental Self—resides in the innermost space of the heart and symbolizes the soul, the air, and the breath. Since ancient times, the soul or the spirit has been identified with breath. *Anima* is the Latin word for soul, breath, and air. The Hebrew word *ruach*, the Arabic word *ruch*, and the Greek *pneuma*, are words that denote both spirit and breath.

The prana in the breath connects the seven chakras, the five elements, and the electrochemical changes that take place in the two hemispheres of the brain. Accumulating prana within the mind and body allows a more complete integration of the physical, mental, and spiritual dimensions within ourselves.

Rhythmic breathing is an ancient technology for uniting our ordinary consciousness with our authentic Self. In the heart and lung center, the pranic energy riding on the air is absorbed directly into the energy of our minds and bodies. The sacred breath, the inspiration of the consciousness of universal intelligence, permeates all of nature. We exist within it, and it within us.

The yantra of the heart chakra is a twelve-petaled lotus the light crimson color of the rising sun (see color plate "Fourth Chakra"). The lotus contains a smoky blue-gray, six-pointed star formed by two interlocking triangles in perfect equilibrium. This six-pointed star, the symbol of air, expresses the energy of the fourth chakra radiating out through all dimensions and directions. The downward-pointing triangle represents the creative energy of Shakti. The upward pointing triangle is Shiva, or ultimate consciousness. This represents the perfect union of the macrocosm with microcosm, male and female, positive and negative, the marriage of the spiritual and material worlds, and the balancing of the three lower chakras with the three highest chakras. Within the hexagon is a downward-pointing triangle. Inside this triangle burns the unflickering eternal flame of our individual soul. This is the All-Shining One, a pure light radiating from the heart chakra. In Catholic traditions, Jesus Christ is often painted with a heart so brilliant it appears as a bright flame.

The bija syllable Yang is the sound of the elemental energy of air and the dimensions of consciousness embodied in the fourth chakra. The elemental quality of air is reflected in the flow of the mind, and is the breath that we all share. An unstable mind is easily distracted, blown here and there by ever changing thoughts. Chanting Yang brings the mind into a one-pointed flow of concentrated awareness.

The black antelope, the power animal of this chakra, is as elusive as the speed of the wind. She is as hard to catch as many of our less-than-conscious thoughts and ideas that shape our reality. Alert and sensitive to each and every sound, she embodies total perceptual awareness.

The primary fears aroused in this chakra are of loneliness, commitment, being unable to protect ourselves emotionally, emotional weakness, and betrayal. Loss of fourth chakra energy can give rise to jealousy, bitterness, anger, hatred, and an inability to forgive others as well as ourselves. The primary strengths to draw on are forgiveness, compassion, dedication, inspiration, hope, trust, and the ability to heal ourselves and others.

Within every one of us resides misconceptions about who we are. We all have traces of dysfunctional self-images, patterns of negative thinking, and painful memories that have accrued through our life experiences. Even though we may recognize these thoughts as unhealthy, until we transform them they can damage our health, relationships, and professional lives. Practicing yoga enables us to begin releasing the wounded aspects of the self that wield authority over our thoughts.

An old French proverb says, "To understand everything is to forgive everything." We free ourselves and heal most quickly through the power of forgiveness. To release the injuries of the past, we must care enough for the priority of our spiritual development to forgive. Through forgiveness, we clear our minds of the control that past wounds have over us. We do it for ourselves and not for those who wounded us, although this process probably helps them as well. Mahatma Gandhi said, "To forgive is not to forget. The merit lies in loving in spite of the vivid knowledge that the one that must be loved is not a friend."[10] Releasing our resentment, anger, and hatred through forgiveness frees the mind. We may find that we do not need to stay in relation to those who continually do hurtful things, even immediate family members. Sometimes the most healing and courageous act is to move on into a life free from conflict and angry emotions.

The spiritual path can be perceived as a crazy and selfish path by the tribal mind. From his family's perspective, the Buddha abandoned them and his position as king in his search for spiritual enlightenment and the realization of compassion and lovingkindness for all beings. True spiritual evolution generally leads one out of the life society expects us to lead. Consider the uproar if government leaders suddenly based all of their decisions on caring for all sentient beings rather than satisfying the desires of the financial powers that put them in office.

The sacred truth of the fourth chakra is that love is the true power that will enable us to attain our goals. While the world assumes that force, might, and violent aggression are the most potent powers on earth, they can never guide our consciousness into the true source of its own power.

Yantra Meditation Instructions for the Fourth Chakra

- Place the Anahata yantra (see color plate "Fourth Chakra") at reading distance with the bindu in the center of the yantra at eye level.
- This yantra is a lotus with twelve petals the color of the red dawn sky. In the center of this lotus is a smoky blue-gray hexagram, the symbol of air.
- Take a seated posture with the spine straight.
- Gaze with a soft focus at the center of the yantra. Keep your eyes focused on the bindu so that you can see the entire yantra.
- Practice the Full Yogic Breath along with Track One on the enclosed CD or on your own. As you do the breathing practice, let your consciousness be drawn into the bindu.
- Practice for five minutes. It is perfectly fine to extend the duration of the meditation on the yantra. ✻

LISTEN TO TRACK 1
Full Yogic Breath

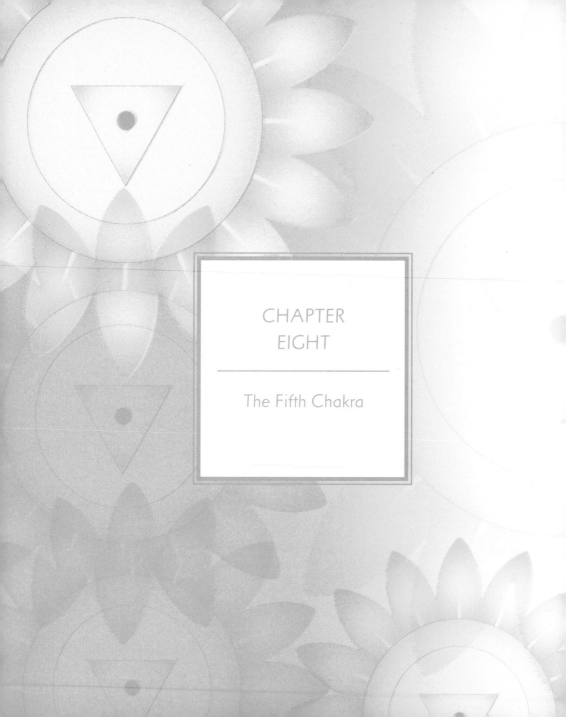

CHAPTER
EIGHT

The Fifth Chakra

Communication Central: Power of Purification

LOCATED IN THE REGION of the throat, Vishuddha chakra is the center of purification, communication, and dreams. When the energy of Kundalini Shakti rises to this chakra, contentment, serenity, and the great gift of detachment develop. The archetypal symbolism, dimensions, and messages of the dream states are understood. The unique power of the fifth chakra is verbalizing and communicating information from all of the other chakras. Vishuddha controls the functioning of the vocal cords and the physical organs of hearing. At the throat center, the thoughts and emotions of the heart convert into audible sound. When Vishuddha is activated, the voice takes on a profound power and beauty, penetrating and vibrationally transforming the hearts of those who hear it.

Vishuddha is the bridge between the chakras of the lower body and the chakra of the brain. In the first four chakras, Shakti manifests as the elements of earth, water, fire, and air. When Shakti reaches the fifth chakra, the elements of the lower chakras are purified and refined as they dissolve into the elemental energy of space. Above Vishuddha, Shakti manifests directly as consciousness.

The geometric yantra of Vishuddha is a lotus with sixteen silvery violet petals (see color plate "Fifth Chakra"). In the center of this lotus is a luminous white circle, which contains a shining translucent triangle. This form represents the energy of *akasha*, or space, connected to the sense perception of hearing and the power of sound. Hang is the seed syllable of space. Within the triangle is a smaller lunar sphere representing the *nada*, the pure cosmic sound reverberating throughout endless space. Meditating on the yantra of this chakra while chanting Hang dissolves the conceptual mind into the purity and vastness of space. The search for solitude in which to pursue spiritual practices is the motivating desire of Vishuddha.

The moon in Vishuddha represents the power of communication without words. Vishuddha tunes in to the thoughts and emotions of people broadcast from near or far, from the past, present, or future. Thoughts, verbal and nonverbal, may be sensed in our gut at Manipura chakra, but they are received in Vishuddha chakra. Vishuddha's awareness of these thoughts is transmitted to the cognitive mind at the sixth chakra, where that information enters into our conscious awareness. On a subtle level, we are intuitively aware of information before we are actually conscious of it. As the chakras are purified and energized, this intuitive perceptual ability expands, becoming clearer and more accurate. We begin to trust our intuition as a legitimate and accurate source of information, accepting its intelligence more rapidly into our conscious minds.

When this center is open, we receive direct messages from the highest levels of consciousness and become a translator of that information. Activating the fifth chakra leads to finding our authentic voice. We develop the ability to express powerful truths in such a way that they can be heard and understood. The ability to communicate creatively and effectively through speaking, writing, singing, music, and dance is the power of the fifth chakra.

Moving from Anahata to Vishuddha, Jung said, "One should even admit that all one's psychical facts have nothing to do with material facts. For instance, the anger which you feel for somebody or something, no matter how justified it is, is not caused by those external things. It is a phenomenon all by itself."[11] He explained that the person you are angry with is really yourself. You project yourself into him, your shadow appears in him, and that makes you angry. He went on to say, "We are perhaps identical even with our own worst enemy. In other words, our worst enemy is perhaps within ourselves."[12]

We understand this when we enter into Vishuddha. We see the world as a projection of our own mind. We recognize the people around us as messengers, or translators of our own psychological condition. Jung tells us, "Whatever befalls you, whatever experience or adventure you have in the external world, is your own experience."[13] The world mirrors our own psyche. The energizing and balancing of the Vishuddha chakra gives us a sense of calm detachment in witnessing the events around us. We are able to understand the role our own consciousness plays in the unfolding of events.

The animal power of the Vishuddha is the elephant that we first saw at Muladhara. In the first chakra, the elephant appears as the substantiality of the earth, the power of consciousness that gives us the ability to survive in the world. At the second chakra, this animal transforms into the makara, the crocodile, a submerged devouring force in the unconscious watery depths of our minds. The power that supported us in our initial drive to consciousness, connecting us to our family and our community, is now the force that we must transcend to survive the explorations of the unconscious. Moving to the third chakra, the animal power appears as the sacrificial ram, and represents not only the sacrifice of our fiery passions, but the strong energy to push forward into change. To be unconscious of our driving passions is the danger. We sacrifice tumultuous passions by becoming conscious of them, releasing their habitual grip on our behavior and moving into emotional freedom. At the fourth chakra, the animal power takes the form of the antelope, an elusive animal that exists lightly on the earth, barely held down by gravity, symbolizing thought and feeling beyond the ego. It is the delicate presence of the soul. At the fifth chakra, the animal power takes its final form, once again as the elephant. At the first chakra, the elephant supported the material reality of the earth; here the ethereal white elephant supports the spatial consciousness of the fifth chakra, purifying our thoughts and mind. At the sixth chakra, the animal power evolves beyond form into the unified organizing power of the cognitive mind.

In the vastness of space at Vishuddha, we get the first glimpse of the metaphysical void of transcendence. This empty, open dimension of being is freed from the constraints of the ego's constant thinking and conceptualizing about personal experiences.

In the void of space, the mind has detached from thought, becoming clear and form-less. It is the vast field of potentiality—unbounded, undefined, and eternal.

The ultimate purpose of yoga is the detachment from conceptualizing thought that obscures the true Self. The mind is withdrawn from all sense objects and then detached from even the most subtle of thoughts. By releasing the activity of the mind and allowing the emptiness of space to fill awareness, the authentic Self begins to be revealed.

The Vishuddha chakra is the great void of space whose comprehension can be a fearful and overwhelming experience. Here we must exist without defining the self in relationship to anything else. Once we have surrendered to and released the fear of being undefinable, a sense of freedom and nonattachment to the world and to the results of actions develops. Kundalini Shakti can then flow upward and into the sixth chakra. At Ajna chakra, the highest expansion of intellectual powers and meditative states of awareness is reached. The only remaining desire is for complete union with the ultimate awareness of the seventh chakra, the Sahasrara. Kundalini's progressive ascension of energy through the six chakras culminates in an electrifying union with the ultimate source of everything in the Sahasrara.

Yantra Meditation Instructions for the Fifth Chakra

• Place the Vishuddha yantra (see color plate "Fifth Chakra") at reading distance with the bindu in the center of the yantra at eye level.
• This yantra is a lotus with sixteen smoky gray-violet petals. In the center of this lotus is a translucent full moon. Within the full moon is an even more translucent downward-pointing triangle.
• Take a seated posture with the spine straight.
• Gaze with a soft focus at the center of the yantra. Keep your eyes focused on the bindu so that you can see the entire yantra.

LISTEN TO TRACK 1
Full Yogic Breath

• Practice the Full Yogic Breath along with Track One on the enclosed CD or on your own. As you do the breathing practice, let your consciousness be drawn into the bindu.
• Practice for five minutes. It is perfectly fine to extend the duration of the meditation on the yantra. 🌼

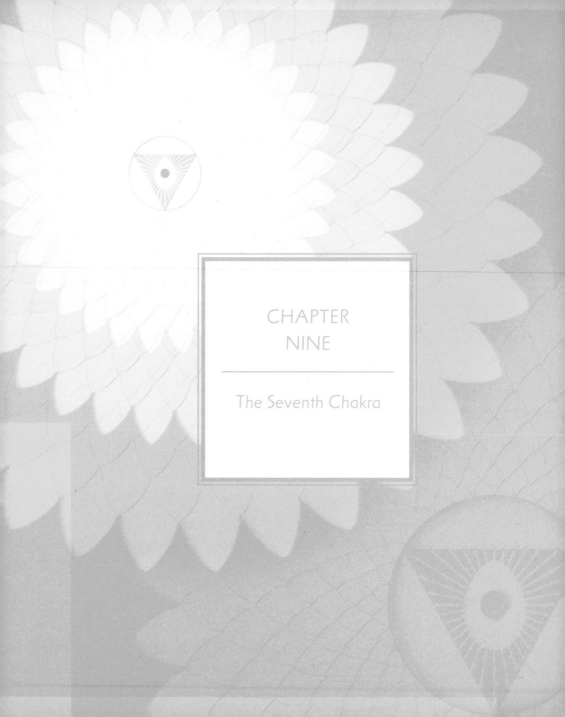

CHAPTER NINE

The Seventh Chakra

Infinite Intelligence: Unification of the Mind

THE CROWN CHAKRA, Sahasrara, is the symbol of the transcendental state of absolute existence, ultimate knowledge, and bliss—the super-conscious state of thought-free awareness. This seventh dimension is the original consciousness, the eternal quality of the universe saturating reality. Here, Kundalini Shakti will unite with Shiva in a sacred marriage, giving birth to the spiritual unity of the chakras. The chakras will then transform from centers of response and habitual reactions into cohesive powerhouses of unified energy. At this point, anything can be accomplished; anything becomes possible.

At the sixth chakra, there is still an experience of the individual self separate from a conception of God, or the ultimate source of reality. There is still the yearning for complete union with the divine. When Kundalini Shakti reunites with the original source of creation in Sahasrara, we understand that there never was anything missing, never was a separation, only obscurities of the mind concealing the truth of Oneness. The crown chakra is a spectrum of Oneness, an extended field of consciousness, the source and energy of everything. All of the lower chakras are experienced simultaneously in this highest state of awareness, leading to the experience of the totality of the Self.

The Sahasrara is not actually a chakra, even though it is often referred to as one. The chakras, as individual dimensions of interrelated thought and emotion, belong to the domain of the mind and body. Sahasrara does not belong to the mind and body, but is experienced just above the crown of the head. A mediating point between the psyche and higher realities, it is the culmination of the evolution of Kundalini Shakti as she rises up the sushumna through each chakra. When Kundalini shoots from the top of the sushumna through the crown of the head into the Sahasrara, we merge with the field of infinite intelligence.

The power of each chakra resides not in itself but in Sahasrara. The chakras function as switches to areas of our consciousness, while the generator of the energies that power the chakras is the Sahasrara. The crown chakra is an all-pervading mind that can operate simultaneously through all the dimensions of awareness embodied in the chakras and reorganize the functioning of each chakra. When awakened, the chakras become perfectly integrated into the totality of the psyche, reorganizing the structure of our energy, thoughts, and emotions. The fields of information of all outer and inner experiences are efficiently correlated and accessible. The elemental energy of Sahasrara is primordial consciousness itself, which permeates all dimensions of reality. Uniting the information and awareness of all the chakras in the consciousness of Sahasrara results in the transcendental unification of the Self.

A lotus with 1,000 white petals, representing 1,000 nadis, or lines of energy, emanating from this center symbolizes the Sahasrara chakra. But in reality, the petals, the nadis, are of infinite number, each humming at the frequency of one of the fifty bija mantras of the Sanskrit alphabet, generating a great symphony of Aum. In the center of the endless number of humming and glowing petals is the full moon shining brilliantly. Within the full moon glows a radiant triangle containing the supreme bindu, the compacted energy of the universe, in the form of a golden, pulsing cosmic egg. This is the seat of the mantra *Hangsah*, which is Shiva in union with Kundalini Shakti—the brilliant luminosity of the divine, the source of the pulse. This is the sacred mind described by all traditions as heaven, God, self-realization, enlightenment, *samadhi*, or *nirvana*—an experience of ten million rays of lustrous humming light.

Enlightenment, nirvana, or *samadhi* are descriptions of super-conscious awareness. In the first five chakras, there is the sensual awareness of smell, taste, sight, touch, and sound. At the sixth chakra, there is the mental awareness of time, space, and object. At the seventh chakra, there is the super-conscious awareness of the Self as the Infinite.

Our mind is a stream of consciousness, transforming and evolving from one stage into the next. The seven stages of the chakras form a connecting ladder between the energies of earth at the first chakra and heaven at the seventh chakra. This is Jacob's Ladder, leading from the material plane to the heavenly realm of pure consciousness. In order to be spiritually, emotionally, and mentally whole, the ladder must be complete. Each chakra must be opened, balanced, and energized to reach the clear mind of our original nature, to reunite Shakti with Shiva.

When Kundalini has finished her evolutionary journey of separation and returns to union with Shiva at the Sahasrara chakra, all individuality dissolves into *Sat-Chit-Ananda*—truth, consciousness, bliss. Final union is achieved with our own true Self. Everything is realized.

Yantra Meditation Instructions for the Seventh Chakra

- Place the Sahasrara yantra, on page 64 at reading distance with the bindu in the center of the yantra at eye level.
- This yantra is a thousand-petaled white lotus. In the center is the full moon shining brilliantly. Inside the circular moon is a lightning-like luminous triangle. Within the triangle is the void, the supreme bindu, the compacted pulsing consciousness of all that is, all that ever was, all that will ever be, in the form of a pulsing, golden, cosmic egg.
- Take a seated posture with the spine straight.
- Gaze with a soft focus at the center of the yantra. Keep your eyes focused on the bindu so that you can see the entire yantra.
- Practice the Full Yogic Breath along with Track One on the enclosed CD or on your own. As you do the breathing practice, let your consciousness be drawn into the bindu.

LISTEN TO TRACK 1
Full Yogic Breath

- Practice for five minutes. It is perfectly fine to extend the duration of the meditation on the yantra. ✿

CHAPTER
TEN

Purification Practices for the Chakras

NOW THAT YOU HAVE explored the individual chakra system as a power map of the structure of consciousness, you are ready to begin practicing the techniques designed to balance and energize all of the chakras. As you do these practices, the samskaras that cause you to react in habitual patterns are dissolved, leaving the mind calmly energized and in a state of concentrated awareness.

Through consistent practice, you will gather and store pranic energy, enabling you to harmonize the chakras and to clear the blockages from the nadis. Practicing regularly is more important than practicing a lot every now and then. In addition, it is highly recommended that you incorporate into your schedule a yoga practice of asanas, which prepares the body for the techniques we are about to learn.

Tips for Practice
• Practice on an empty stomach.
• Find a quiet, uncluttered space where others or the phone will not interrupt you.

- Sit with spine erect; do not lie down. If you can sit on the floor in any of the classic yoga postures, that would be ideal. You may also sit on the floor against a wall, with legs outstretched, or in a chair with a straight back. It is important that the spine is straight in all of the practices. The following practices are fully guided on the accompanying CD. Read through the information on the guided sessions before beginning to enhance the learning process and to be fully informed about contraindicated conditions.

Full Yogic Breath—Foundation for Many Pranayama Techniques

LISTEN TO TRACK 1
Full Yogic Breath

BENEFITS This basic breathing practice maximizes inhalation and exhalation, increases oxygen intake, corrects poor breathing habits, and develops conscious breath awareness. It improves lymphatic drainage from the lower part of the lungs; massages the organs that surround the diaphragm (the liver, intestines, and stomach); and calms nervous tension and emotional upset.

Take a seated position with the spine erect. Exhale completely. Inhale slowly through the nose, deep into the abdomen, feeling the diaphragm contract while the stomach expands, filling the lowest lobes of the lungs. Continue inhaling into the upper chest, feeling the ribcage expanding and the middle part of the lungs filling. Inhale a little more, feeling the expansion in the upper portion of the lungs at the base of the neck. Pause, then exhale with the lower neck and shoulders relaxing, followed by the ribcage relaxing and contracting downward and inward. The diaphragm relaxes upward, followed by a contraction of the abdominal area to completely empty the lungs. Practice a round of five full yogic breaths.

Yogic Eye Exercises and the Eye Lock, or Shambhavi Mudra

LISTEN TO TRACK 2
Eye Lock

BENEFITS These exercises relax, revitalize, and strengthen the muscles of the eyes; release stress and anger, and develop concentration and mental stability.

CONTRAINDICATIONS The following conditions would prohibit practice of eye exercises except under the directions of a medical professional: Diseases of the eyes such as glaucoma, cataracts, retinal detachment, or conjunctivitis. Obtain medical guidance if you have had lens implants, laser eye surgery, or other eye operations. Do not wear glasses or contact lenses while performing these exercises. At the first sign of strain, release the exercise and relax the eyes.

Yogic Eye Exercises
Sit with the spine erect. Hold the right arm straight out in front of the nose, making a fist with the right hand, point the thumb upward. Focus both eyes on the tip of the thumb. Bend the arm and slowly bring the thumb to the center of the forehead, keeping the eyes focused on the thumb tip. Pause and slowly straighten the arm, continuing to gaze at the thumb tip. This is one round. As a beginner, you can do five rounds, if you do not feel strain.

On the next round, synchronize moving your thumb with the exhalation and inhalation. Hold the right fist straight out with the thumb pointing upward. Focus both eyes on the tip of the thumb. To begin, exhale and then inhale, bending the arm and slowly bringing the thumb to the middle of the forehead. Keep the eyes focused on the tip of the thumb. Pause and then exhale slowly, straightening the arm, continuing to gaze at the thumb tip. Pause and then inhale, bending the arm and slowly bringing the thumb to the tip of the nose. Pause and then exhale, straightening the arm while continuing to gaze at the thumb. Do a total of five rounds synchronized with the breath if that is comfortable for the eyes.

When you finish, rub both palms together until they feel hot. Then cover your closed eyes with your warmed palms, absorbing the healing warmth into the eyes.

The Eye Lock, or Shambhavi Mudra
The practice of *Shambhavi Mudra* circulates energy that normally flows out through the eyes back into the sixth chakra. The sixth chakra is stimulated, encouraging the development of paranormal vision and super-conscious perceptions. This practice strengthens and relaxes the eye muscles, the entire face, and the rest of the body.

With the spine erect and head upright, close and relax the eyes. Now open the eyes and look straight ahead. With the eyes only, look upward and inward, at the point between the eyebrows. Gently keep the eyes focused in that position without straining. At the first sensation of strain, relax your eyes, look straight ahead, and then close them. Gradually, the eyes can be held comfortably in this position for longer lengths of time. As you begin to develop the muscles that move and focus your eyes, you can move to the next step of synchronizing the breath with the movement of the eyes.

Close and relax your eyes. Open the eyes and look straight ahead. Exhale and then inhale slowly as the eyes raise and focus on the point between the eyebrows. Gently keep them focused in that position while retaining the breath for a few seconds. Now begin to exhale, and lower the gaze back to straight ahead. Do a series of five rounds. When you finish, rub both palms together and then cover your closed eyes with your warmed palms.

As the nerves and muscles of the eyes strengthen and habitual tension around the eyes is released, you can do this practice with the eyes closed. As you strengthen the muscles that focus your eyes, you will be able to hold the eye lock for longer periods of time. As you build endurance, you will not keep the eyes synchronized with the breath. You will breathe normally as you hold the lock.

Breath of Fire, or Kapalbhati

LISTEN TO TRACK 3
Breath of Fire

This energizing pranayama should be done before meditation.

BENEFITS *Kapalbhati* purifies the frontal lobes of the brain by rapid breathing through the nose with an emphasis on exhalation. In Sanskrit, *kapal* means the "cranium" or "forehead." *Bhati* is "light," "splendor," "perception," or "knowledge." This practice invigorates the entire brain, awakening the dormant centers that are responsible for subtle perception. In normal breathing, the emphasis is on the inhale. Kapalbhati reverses this process, making the exhalation active and inhalation passive. In a normal inhalation, the fluid around the brain is compressed, causing the brain to contract slightly. This cerebrospinal fluid is decompressed during exhalation, and the brain very minutely expands. In the forced exhalation of Kapalbhati, this massaging and stimulating effect on the brain is enhanced. More carbon dioxide is expelled, cleansing the respiratory system and nasal passages, and removing impurities of the blood. This benefits those with emphysema, asthma, bronchitis, and tuberculosis. Kapalbhati purifies ida and pingala nadis, energizing the mind for mental work, relieving drowsiness, and creating a feeling of exhilaration. In addition, Kapalbhati helps prepare women for childbirth.

CONTRAINDICATIONS If you experience dizziness or faintness, stop and sit calmly until your breathing returns to normal. The following conditions would prohibit practice of Kapalbhati except under the supervision of an experienced teacher or medical professional: high blood pressure, history of stroke, heart disease, epilepsy, hernia, and gastric ulcer.

Take a seated posture with the spine and head erect. Place the hands on the thighs. Do not rock the body with the forceful exhalation of the breath. This is an abdominal breath; the upper part of the lungs is not activated. The strong contraction of the abdominal muscles causes the short rhythmic expulsion of breath. The inhalation is a natural result of the forceful exhalation.

Close the eyes and relax the body. Practice ten inhalations and exhalations at the rate of about one per second. Inhale though the nose deep into the expanding abdomen, and then exhale with a forceful contraction of the abdominal muscles. At the end of the ten breaths, the last exhale is slower and completely empties the lungs. Then take a full yogic breath in and out. Breathe normally for a minute before beginning the next round. As a beginner, you can do up to five rounds of ten breaths. Gradually increase the speed and number of breaths until reaching a total of 120 exhalations per round.

Alternate Nostril Breathing, or Nadi Shodhana

In Sanskrit, *shodhana* means "to purify," and *Nadi Shodhana* purifies the energy channels in the body, balancing the flow of Shakti in the ida and pingala nadis. This causes prana to flow through the main sushumna channel, influencing all of the chakras, particularly the sixth chakra.

LISTEN TO TRACK 4
Alternate Nostril Breathing

BENEFITS Nadi Shodhana cleans the blood of toxins, and nourishes the body by supplying extra oxygen. Very productive for those engaged in mental work, this practice increases concentration and clarity while lowering anxiety and stress. It also is helpful for overcoming insomnia.

To practice Nadi Shodhana, use the full yogic breath and always breathe in through the left nostril to begin the rounds. Sit with the spine erect and hold your right hand in front of your face. Fold in your middle and index finger with the thumb, keeping the ring and the little finger extended. Exhale and close the right nostril with your thumb. Breathe in deeply and slowly through the left nostril. Pause and then close the left nostril with your ring finger and open the right nostril. Exhale completely and slowly through the right nostril. Pause. Breathe in through the right nostril and then pause. Now close the right nostril with your thumb and open the left nostril. Exhale through the left nostril. This is one round. Practice five rounds to start, and then in future sessions, work up to ten as quickly as you feel comfortable.

Always breathe in through the left nostril to begin the rounds, and end rounds by exhaling through the left nostril. Starting and ending the rounds by breathing through the right nostril affects a different hemisphere of the brain along with different nadis in the body, and is not as beneficial for yogic purposes.

The Perineum Lock, or Mula Bandha

LISTEN TO TRACK 5
Perineum Lock

Mula Bandha is an energy-charging practice. *Bandha*, in Sanskrit, means "to hold," "tighten, lock, stop," or "to redirect." The bandhas rejuvenate and revitalize the body, keeping it healthy and youthful by redirecting the prana into the sushumna nadi to help awaken Kundalini Shakti. Mula Bandha is actually the contraction of the center point of the perineum, a group of muscles extending the entire length of the pelvic floor, containing the rectum as well as the urinary and sexual organs. The point of the perineum contracted is midway between the rectum and the sexual organs.

To locate the perineum, press your finger midway between the genitals and rectum. Develop awareness of the pelvic floor as a muscular sheath stretching from the tailbone to the pelvic bone wrapping around the urethra, vagina or root of the penis, and the rectum in a figure eight pattern. In the beginning you can contract the muscles as if you were trying to stop urinating, contracting both the genitals and the sphincter muscles. As you practice you will gain more awareness and control, eventually contracting or pulling upwards mainly at the midpoint location of the perineum.

When contracting and then releasing a group of muscles, a subtle process of unlocking and releasing of mental and pranic energies occurs, leading to both physical and mental relaxation. Mula Bandha contracts the Muladhara chakra, the seat of Kundalini and the kanda that sends energy up the sushumna to Ajna chakra, influencing all of the chakras. As the perineum is contracted, the kanda, the root of the entire nadi system, contracts, transmitting bursts of prana throughout the nadis and chakras—clearing away blockages or psychic knots of anxieties, tensions, repressions, and unresolved conflicts in our unconscious.

BENEFITS The most immediate effect of this practice is a deep sense of mental relaxation and peace, relieving stress, anxiety, tension, depression, and panic attacks. Physically contracting the perineum maintains hormonal balance; stimulates and regulates the pelvic nerves; tones the urogenital and excretory organs; and stabilizes the menstrual cycle. Mula Bandha slows respiration, inducing relaxation and calmness; lowers blood pressure, relaxing the heart; and soothes the brain and nervous system. Peristalsis is also stimulated, helping to overcome constipation. In preparing for childbirth, this practice maintains elasticity of the vaginal muscles, and after childbirth assists in retoning stretched muscles. It is useful for treating urinary incontinence and uterine prolapse. During menopause, this practice rebalances hormonal changes, helping to prevent high blood pressure, depression, lethargy, and irritability. In men, it helps prevent inguinal hernias.

CONTRAINDICATIONS The following conditions would prohibit practice of Mula Bandha except under the directions of an experienced teacher or medical professional: high blood pressure, heart conditions, high intracranial pressure (excessive pressure in the brain), vertigo, amenorrhea (the absence of menstrual bleeding in females of reproductive age), and hemorrhoids.

Take a seated posture. Focus attention on the perineum. Contract the perineum and forcibly draw it upward, then relax. Contract the perineum ten times with maximum contraction and then total relaxation as evenly and rhythmically as possible while continuing to breathe normally. This is considered one round of ten contractions.

Now synchronize the contractions with the breath. Focus on the perineum, inhaling deeply. Hold the breath, contract the perineum, and then hold. Now release the perineum, exhale, and relax. Contract ten times synchronized with the breath to complete one round of contractions. You can work up to thirty contractions per round. Finish by sitting calmly with eyes closed, allowing your breathing to return to normal.

Fixed Gazing at One Point, or Trataka

BENEFITS Trataka stabilizes awareness in the sixth chakra, strengthening the eyes; concentrating the mind; improving memory; and relieving anxiety, depression, and insomnia. By limiting the sense

LISTEN TO TRACK 6
Fixed Gazing at One Point

perception of sight to one object only, the mind is "turned off," allowing suppressed thoughts and experiences to be recognized and released.

CONTRAINDICATIONS Epileptics should not practice Trataka by gazing at a flame. Instead, use a stationary object such as a dot, a yantra, or a sculpture.

Sit with the spine erect, in a dark room with no moving air to disturb the flame of the candle. Place the candle at eye level at a distance of two feet. Close the eyes and let the eyes, face, and body relax. Now, open the eyes and stare directly at the brightest part of the flame, just above the tip of the wick. Try not to blink. Let the flame completely fill your awareness, allowing all thoughts to subside. When the eyes become tired or water, close them and look for the afterimage of the flame in your mind's eye. Concentrate on this image as you did the flame, until it fades from your inner vision. Continue by alternately gazing at the candle until the eyes tire, and then closing the eyes and watching the mental image of the flame. Initially, practice Trataka for several minutes, gradually increasing the duration of the gaze until you have reached ten minutes. Try to keep from blinking even when the eyes begin to water. This cleanses the tear ducts and releases a natural antiseptic, *lysozyme*, which keeps the eyes infection-free. When you finish, rub both palms together, and then cover your closed eyes with your warmed palms.

Purification of the Chakras Meditation

LISTEN TO TRACK 7
Purification of the Chakras

This meditation is based on traditional *Bhuta Shuddhi* meditations, which purify the elemental energies of the chakras. It combines yantra practice with the chanting of the seed mantras. As you move your awareness through the chakras, gaze at the corresponding illustration of the individual chakras.

Ideal Practice Schedule

After several months of gaining endurance and concentration, this is the ideal practice schedule to follow daily:
• Eye Lock, or Shambhavi Mudra, five minutes.
• Breath of Fire, or Kapalbhati for two rounds of 120 breaths, five minutes.
• Alternate Nostril Breathing, or Nadi Shodhana using full yogic breath for ten rounds. five minutes.

- Perineum Lock, or Mula Bandha. Ten contractions using the full yogic breath with breath retention, five minutes.
- Fixed Gazing at One Point, or Trataka, ten minutes.
- Purification of the Chakras Meditation, ten minutes.

Doing all of the practices in one session takes sixty-five minutes. This is the most powerful way to do the practices, but the material can be broken into two sessions, if necessary. Do the first six guided practices as one session, and the Purification of the Chakras Meditation as a separate session. To prepare for the Purification of the Chakras Meditation, do Kapalbhati for two rounds, followed by five minutes of Trataka to settle the mind. It is important to develop a schedule that you can maintain.

These powerful yogic practices reorganize, revitalize, and transform the energetic structure of the body and mind. The entire nadi and chakra system can be cleansed of blockages, allowing a free flow of energy, helping to rejuvenate the body and clear the mind. The more you practice, the more centered and powerful your concentration becomes. The more prana you accumulate, the more magnetic you become, the more completely your mind functions, and the more energy you will have to dissolve the obstructions that are blocking the full manifestation of your ultimate Self. ✤

CHAPTER ELEVEN

Lineage

I WANT TO EXPRESS my tremendous gratitude to my teachers, as well as provide a brief historical background of the classical sources of our knowledge of the chakras. My primary yoga teacher has been Yogiraj V. Subrahmanya Bua, whose guru was Swami Sivananda Saraswati, founder of the Divine Life Society in India. The books of another student of Swami Sivananda, Swami Satyananda Saraswati of the Bihar School of Yoga in Munger, India, have greatly expanded my understanding of the practices I learned directly from Swami Bua. I also offer heartfelt appreciation to Baba Hari Dass and his senior students at Mount Madonna in Watsonville, California, where I received my yoga teacher training certification. My qigong master, Wei Lun Huang, greatly illuminated the movement of qi in the body for me. My Japanese tea master Hisashi Yamada Sensei's quiet sense of contentment, calmness, and happiness in teaching us to make a bowl of tea informs my everyday thoughts. I benefited immensely from the Shambhala Training meditation program, created by Chögyam Trungpa Rinpoche, completing undergraduate, graduate, and Warrior's Assembly, including two month-long retreats of shamata practice, one under the supervision of Tai Situ Rinpoche, who I took refuge and bodhisattva vows with. Finally, thanks to

Charlotte Vandegrift, with whom I studied Isometric Muscle Rebalancing, the flow of energy through the meridians, and much more. All of these teachers have taught me about the flow of consciousness in the mind and body. I have been very fortunate in my life to have such great teachers.

The material presented in this book is based on the system Swami Sivananda Saraswati taught, and was passed on by his students, Swami Bua and Swami Satyananda Saraswati. This system is similar to the one we studied with Baba Hari Dass and his senior students, but with differences. Puzzled over some of the differing illustrations of the energy channels in the body depicted in various eighteenth and nineteenth century manuscripts from India, I had the opportunity to ask Baba Hari Dass which one was right. He explained that one was Vedic and one was Tantric, not commenting on which was correct, although the system we learned at his center falls under the Tantric description. With further research, I came to understand that I was seeing illustrations of different meditation practices from different traditions. At this point in my understanding, I believe the main energy channels can flow in different patterns based on the meditation practice we are doing. The channels can shift routes based on our concentrated mental perception of their pathways.

Even within the traditions originating in India, there are many different systems of understanding the energetic body and the chakras. These systems cannot be correlated: they differ in the total number of chakras, the number of petals, the colors assigned to the yantra of each chakra, the main mantra seed sounds, and the goddesses and gods that occupy the chakras. Some systems incorporate the elemental energies, animal powers, deities, and geometric forms, and others do not.

The earliest references to the nadis and prana appear in the earlier Upanishads thought to have been written in the seventh to eighth centuries BCE, or perhaps far earlier. The later Upanishads, probably composed between the second century BCE and second century CE, have the first references to Tantric concepts of mantras, chakras, and elemental energies.

Some time between the ninth and the twelfth centuries CE, the Natha Siddha yogis Gorakhnatha and Matsyendranatha founded a sect, based on hatha yoga practices, that had a tremendous influence on the development of yoga. Matsyendranatha wrote the *Kaulajnana Nirnaya*, describing an eight-fold chakra system. Each of the eight chakras have eight petals. There are no geometric forms, animal powers, or gods or goddesses in these depictions, and the seed syllable for each chakra is different from the system in this program. Around the fifteenth century, the scholar yogi Swatmarama, influenced by the Natha Siddhas, wrote the *Hatha Yoga Pradipika*, a very powerful compilation of yoga practices central to the teachings of Swami Shivananda and his students.

In 1557, a Bengali yogi Purnananda wrote the *Sat-Cakra-Nirupana*, a Tantric treatise on the seven chakras. Sir John Woodroffe, an English judge living in India in the early 1900s, translated the text into English. Under the pseudonym of Arthur Avalon, he included it in his book, *The Serpent Power*, published in 1919. This text has been the primary source of information on the chakras for most Western students of yoga.

In 1932, the psychoanalyst Carl G. Jung held a seminar on the psychology of Kundalini Yoga based on the *Sat-Cakra-Nirupana*. For Jung, this text provided a model for understanding the developmental phases of higher consciousness. From his wide knowledge of the world's traditions of mythology and religion, he approached the chakras as archetypes and symbols of transformations of inner experiences in the process of individuation. This information was preserved in the book, *The Psychology of Kundalini Yoga: Notes of the Seminar*.

Other chakra systems have grown out of the Vedic or Tantric traditions. In the nineteenth century, Huzur Swamiji Maharaj drew from Hindu, Tantric, Sufi, and Sikh traditions, creating a new tradition, Sant Mat, with many followers in India today. This system has six lower chakras and six higher chakras. There are also Tibetan Buddhist systems that use five, seven, or ten chakras. In addition, the Taoist system of meridians and dan tiens has some similarities as well as substantial differences. Hiroshi Motoyama, who holds doctorates in psychology and philosophy, correlates these two systems in his book *The Theories of the Chakras*, which has a foreword by Swami Satyananda Saraswati.

The Theosophical Society, founded in 1875, is a tradition in which the main teachers and thinkers blended clairvoyant information with concepts of Hinduism, Buddhism, the Egyptian Hermetic philosophy, Taoism, Neoplatonism, Kabbalism, Freemasonry, Rosicrucianism, and Spiritualism. In 1927, the Theosophist C.W. Leadbeater wrote *The Chakras*, a book that greatly influenced the contemporary "new age" view of the chakras.

In 1976, the North Indian teacher Harish Johari published *Chakras: Energy Centers of Transformation*, correlating traditional information on the chakras with Western scientific studies on the brain.

In 1977, Christopher Hill published a book, *Nuclear Evolution: Discovery of the Rainbow Body*, in which he correlated the chakras to the rainbow spectrum of light, with red representing the first chakra, orange, the second chakra, and so forth. This has so firmly caught on that almost every book written by a Western author since that date has used the rainbow spectrum in describing the chakras. Yet this correlation does not exist in the traditions from India. Furthermore, the "new age" philosophy of the chakras is strongly influenced by the concept of healing ourselves and developing the ability to heal others through understanding the energetics behind the chakras. This is quite different from the original Tantric purpose of meditating on the chakras as a means of dissolving samskaras and obstacles blocking the union of the individual self with the Divine source of consciousness.

The concept of the chakras as a system of understanding our consciousness has taken on new levels of meaning not apparent in the traditions from India. However, it is clear that traditions have evolved considerably even within India, and that we adjust information to fit our perception of reality, our needs, and the evolution that we are going through as a species. The structure of the chakras is an evolving system of understanding who and what we really are. Traditionally, all knowledge of the chakras originally appeared to advanced yogic practitioners during meditation. In these meditative states of awareness, the practitioners could see the energetic structure of the mind and body. The most talented became teachers and passed this knowledge and wisdom on to their students, contributing to the evolution of the understanding of consciousness. Every one of these teachers has said that all of this vast wisdom is available to anyone who practices correctly with commitment, discipline, and devotion. The path that led me to the teachers that have given me a means to understanding my mind and my life began with the book on yoga I received as a teenager. This motivated me to write this book, and to think carefully about what information and practices to include. In this program, you will find a tried and true technology for understanding the energy structure of your electromagnetic being, and giving you traditional practices for awakening the dimensions of consciousness contained in the chakras. These arts of self-understanding and self-transformation will help you to develop your own authentic voice, purpose, and path in life, leading to the ultimate goal of Self-realization. My own life has been immeasurably enriched by the brilliance of these teachings. It is my greatest pleasure to share the wisdom and grace of this tradition with you. ☀

1 "We still have to be polite to people to avoid the explosions of Manipura." Carl G. Jung, ed., Sonu Shamdasani, *The Psychology of Kundalini Yoga: Notes of the Seminar* (Princeton: Princeton University Press, 1996), p. 41.

2 "She is beautiful like a chain of lightning ..." *Sat-Cakra-Nirupana* quote, Arthur Avalon (Sir John Woodroffe), *The Serpent Power: The Secrets of Tantric and Shaktic Yoga* (New York: Dover Publications, Inc., 1974), p. 328.

3 "The very first demand of a mystery cult always has been to go into water ..." Carl G. Jung, ed., Sonu Shamdasani, *The Psychology of Kundalini Yoga: Notes of the Seminar* (Princeton: Princeton University Press, 1996), p. 16.

4 He spoke of the second chakra as, "the mandala of baptism..." Ibid, p. 17.

5 "Svadhisthana is made up of all ..." S.M. Roney-Dougal, *On a Possible Psychophysiology of the Yogic Chakra System* (Part I), electronic work posted on Swami Satyananda Saraswati's website: http://www.yogamag.net/archives/2000/3may00/chakra1.shtml (accessed February 1, 2004).

6 "According to a provocative insight by Paul MacLean, the higher functions of the brain evolved in three successive stages." Carl Sagan, *Cosmos* (New York: Ballantine, 1985), p. 228.

7 "The soul does not mate ..." From a lesson with Baba Hari Dass at the yoga teacher training intensive, June 2002, at Mt. Madonna. I was present in this session and heard this exchange myself.

8 "... how consciousness came to pass ..." Carl G. Jung, ed., Sonu Shamdasani, *The Psychology of Kundalini Yoga: Notes of the Seminar* (Princeton: Princeton University Press, 1996), p. 30.

9 Manipura's function is to be "aggressive: to conquer, to consume ..." Joseph Campbell, *Transformations of Myth through Time* (New York: Harper & Row, 1990), pgs. 159-160.

10 "To forgive is not to forget ..." Mahatma Ghandi. *The Official Mahatma Gandhi eArchive & Reference Library*, Mahatma Gandhi Foundation, India, electronic work: http://www.mahatma.org.in/quotes/quotes.jsp?link=qt (accessed February 1, 2004).

11 "One should even admit that all one's psychical facts ..." Carl G. Jung, ed., Sonu Shamdasani, *The Psychology of Kundalini Yoga: Notes of the Seminar* (Princeton: Princeton University Press, 1996), p. 49.

12 "We are perhaps identical ..." Carl G. Jung, ed., Sonu Shamdasani, *The Psychology of Kundalini Yoga: Notes of the Seminar* (Princeton: Princeton University Press, 1996), p. 49.

13 "Whatever befalls you ..." Carl G. Jung, ed., Sonu Shamdasani, *The Psychology of Kundalini Yoga: Notes of the Seminar* (Princeton: Princeton University Press, 1996), p. 50.

Ajna aa-gyah. The sixth chakra, located at the medulla oblongata, at the top of the spine, in the center of the brain, Command Central.

Akasha ah-kahsh(a). Space, ether, the elemental energy of the fifth chakra.

Anahata a-nah-hut(a). The unstruck sound, the fourth chakra at the heart center.

Atman aht-mah(n). Highest reality, the supreme consciousness, the individual soul.

Aum ohng. The sound of creation, the primordial mantra.

Bandha bun-dh(a). A posture which creates a psycho-muscular energy lock, controlling and redirecting the flow of prana, locking it into a particular part of the body.

Bhuta Shuddhi bhoot(a)-shoodh-dhi. *Bhuta* means "elements", *shuddhi* means "purification", bhuta shuddhi is a purification of the five elements, earth, water, fire, air, and space.

Bija Mantra bee-j(a) mahn-truh. Seed or basic mantra, a transcendental sound and transformative sound, one of the fifty sounds that make up the energy of Kundalini Shakti.

Bindu bin-doo. The supremely compacted and concentrated point of immense conscious power. It is the sum total of the potential of the universe.

Chakra chak-ruh. The "ch" is pronounced like the "ch" in church, not like the "sh" in shock. Circle, wheel, matrix of energy. The pranic centers, the intersections of the nadis within the body that oversee specific physiological and psychic functions.

Chitta chi-ta. Perceptive mind or individual consciousness, including the unconscious and subconscious dimensions of the mind. Its functions are said to be thinking, memory, attention, concentration, and inquiry.

Hang hung. Bija syllable representing the energy of space at the fifth chakra.

Hangsah hung-suh. Mantra associated with the crown chakra.

Ida i-daah. One of the three major nadis running on the left side of the spine from the first chakra to the sixth chakra, through which mental energy or chitta flows. Controls mental processes.

Kanda kahn-da. The bulb-shaped root of the nadis, said to be three inches wide by nine inches long, originating in the first chakra but extending up to the third chakra. Sometimes texts locate it in the first chakra, and sometimes in the third.

Kapalbhati ka-pahl-bhah-tee. The first *a* is short. Pranayama practice that purifies the frontal section of the brain by rapid breathing through the nostrils, emphasizing the exhalation.

Kundalini Shakti koon-duh-lee-ni shahk-tee. The divine cosmic Power-Consciousness, the human spiritual energy and capacity which lies dormant at the first chakra. This energy must be aroused and caused to ascend through the sushumna, piercing and awakening each chakra, culminating in a grand union with ultimate consciousness at the crown chakra.

Lang lung. Bija syllable representing the energy of the earth element at the first chakra.

Mani Padma ma-ni pad-ma. The Jeweled Lotus, another name for the Manipura chakra.

Manipura ma-ni-poor(a). The Jeweled City at the Navel of Reality, the third chakra.

Mantra man-tra. A subtle transcendental and transformative sound.

Mudra moo-drah. Physical, mental, and psychic position or attitude that controls, focuses, and channels pranic energy within the mind and body.

Mula Bandha mool(a) bun-dh(a). Contraction of the perineum, stimulates Muladhara chakra and helps awaken Kundalini Shakti.

Muladhara moo-lah-dhahr(a). The first chakra, the Root Support.

Nabhi Padma nah-bhee pad-ma. The navel lotus, the third chakra, Manipura.

Nada nahd(a). The pure cosmic sound reverberating throughout endless space.

Nada yoga nahd(a) yoh-g(a). Yoga of subtle sound.

Nadi nah-dee. Literally means flow, subtle flow, or channel of prana in the energy body. A pranic line or movement of energy.

Nadi Chakra nah-dee chak-ruh. The nadi system, the force field formed by the nadis distributed throughout the body.

Nadi-Shodhana nah-di shoh-dhan(a). Pranic purification, the purifying breath. Pranayama breathing practice that purifies the nadis by alternate nostril breathing.

Pingala peen-ga-lah. One of the three major nadis, pingala nadi conducts prana shakti, or vital or physical force, and runs on the right side of the spine from the first chakra to the sixth chakra. Associated with the worldly realm of experience and externalized perception.

Prana prahn(a). The vital life force that permeates and sustains creation, the life force in the body. On the bioenergetic level, it is comparable to the physical breath of air.

Pranayama prahn-a-yahm(a). A system of controlling, enhancing, and accumulating prana within the body by manipulating the breath. The primary means of purifying the nadis, the chakras, and awakening Kundalini.

Rang rung. Bija syllable representing the sound of fire at Manipura, the third chakra.

Sahasrara sa-has-rahr(a). The crown chakra, which contains all of the lower chakras, and is the threshold between the human realm and higher realms of consciousness.

Samadhi sa-mah-dhee. Culmination and fulfillment of yogic meditation, the state of supramental and super-concentrated consciousness. The mind becomes one with its object of concentration and the highest strata of consciousness.

Samskaras sam-skah-r(a)s, or more accurately, sung-skah-r(a)s. The mental impressions, imprints or archetypes stored in the unconscious dimensions of the chakras.

Sat-Chit-Ananda sat-chit-ah-nun-duh. *Sat* means "truth", "pure", or "existence". *Chit* means "consciousness". *Ananda* means "bliss", "pure unalloyed bliss, ecstasy, the highest state of super consciousness."

Shambhavi Mudra shahm-bha-vee moo-druh. The Eye Lock. The eyes are directed to look at the point between the eyebrows, which induces a concentrated and peaceful state of mind. A process of concentration which transforms external seeing into internal gazing.

Shiva shee-v(a). The original source of yoga: the state of pure consciousness on a cosmic and individual level.

Sushumna shoo-shoom-nah. The main channel running through the spine from the first chakra to the sixth chakra. The carrier of spiritual energy.

Svadisthana svad-his-than(a). One's own abode, the second chakra.

Trataka trah-tak(a). A technique for calming, concentrating, and clearing the mind by gazing at a candle, yantra, or other focusing object.

Upanishads oo-pa-ni-shads. Books of the Vedas containing the realizations of sages concerning reality, the nature of true identity, and individual consciousness. Literally means "to sit down near the guru for teachings."

Vang vung. The sound of the elemental energy of water at the second chakra, Svadisthana.

Vishuddha vi-shoodh-dhuh. The fifth chakra at the throat center, the Center of Purification.

Yang yung. The sound of the elemental energy of air at the fourth chakra, Anahata.

Yantra yan-tra. Precision geometric power diagram representing configurations of consciousness. Concentration on a yantra liberates potential energy and consciousness in the mind.

Yoga yoh-g(a). The state of union between Shiva and Shakti, individual and universal consciousness, body and mind. It is the process of uniting these opposite forces within the mind and body to realize the spiritual essence of awareness and being.

Avalon, Arthur (Sir John Woodroffe). *The Serpent Power: The Secrets of Tantric and Shaktic Yoga*. New York: Dover Publications, 1974. Originally published in 1918, it was one of the earliest English translations of texts illustrating the functioning of the chakras.

Feuerstein, Georg. *Tantra: The Path of Ecstasy*. Boston and London: Shambhala, 1998. Excellent introduction to Tantra.

Goswami, Shyam Sundar. *Layayoga: The Definitive Guide to the Chakras and Kundalini*. Rochester, Vermont: Inner Traditions, International, 1999. Exhaustive reference book on traditional information about the chakras.

Iyengar, B.K.S. *Light on Pranayama: The Yogic Art of Breathing*. New York: Crossroad, 1997. Contemporary master of yoga and pranayama.

Johari, Harish. *Chakras: Energy Centers of Transformation*. Rochester, Vermont: Inner Traditions, International, 1988. A traditional perspective on the chakras combined with Western scientific information on the brain.

Khanna, Madhu. *Yantra: The Tantric Symbol of Cosmic Unity*. Rochester, Vermont: Inner Traditions, International, 2003.

Myss, Caroline. *Anatomy of the Spirit*. New York: Random House, 1996. Contemporary intuitive approach combining and correlating various traditions based on the body's seven centers of spiritual and physical power.

Swami Muktibodhananda under the supervision of Swami Satyananda Saraswati, translator. *Hatha Yoga Pradipika*. Munger, Bihar, India: Bihar School of Yoga, 1985. My hatha yoga bible—this is a great translation. All the books from Bihar School of Yoga are excellent.

Swami Niranjanananda Saraswati. *Prana Pranayama Prana Vidya*. Munger, Bihar, India: Bihar School of Yoga, 1985.

Swami Satyananda Saraswati. *Asana Pranayama Mudra Bandha*. Munger, Bihar, India: Bihar School of Yoga, 1966.

Swami Satyananda Saraswati. *Kundalini Tantra*. Munger, Bihar, India: Bihar School of Yoga, 1984.

Swami Satyasangananda. *Tattwa Shuddhi*. Munger, Bihar, India: Yoga Publications Trust, 1984.

LAYNE REDMOND is an acclaimed drummer, composer, author, mythologist, and a lifelong student of yoga. Redmond teaches workshops and performs internationally, specializing in the small, hand-held frame drums played primarily in the ancient Mediterranean world. She is the author of *When the Drummers Were Women*; was named *Drum!* magazine's 2002 Percussionist of the Year; is one of only two women featured in *Planet Drum*, the book about ethnic drumming by The Grateful Dead drummer Mickey Hart; and was the first woman to have a Signature Series of world percussion instruments with Remo, Inc., one of the world's largest manufacturers of percussion instruments.

SOUNDS TRUE was founded in 1985 by Tami Simon, with a clear vision: to disseminate spiritual wisdom. Located in Boulder, Colorado, Sounds True publishes teaching programs that are designed to educate, uplift, and inspire. With more than 600 titles available, we work with many of the leading spiritual teachers, thinkers, healers, and visionary artists of our time.

For a free catalog, or for more information on audio programs by Layne Redmond, please contact Sounds True via the World Wide Web at www.soundstrue.com, call us toll free at 800-333-9185, or write

The Sounds True Catalog
PO Box 8010
Boulder, CO 80306

CD SESSIONS

1. Full Yogic Breath 4:45

2. Eye Lock 10:45

3. Breath of Fire 11:50

4. Alternate Nostril Breathing 5:38

5. Perineum Lock 8:14

6. Fixed Gazing at One Point 7:05

7. Purification of the Chakras Meditation 27:59